Jumbly Words
and Rights Where
Wrongs Should Be

The Experience of Aphasia
from the Inside

Far Communication Disorders Series

Series Editors: Chris Code and David Rowley, Department of Speech Pathology, Leicester Polytechnic, Leicester, England.

The *Far Communication Disorders Series* aims to provide books in speech and language pathology and therapy for the clinician and student clinician. Each book in the series will aim to be practical, readable and affordable. Currently available and forthcoming titles include:

Parents, Families, and the Stuttering Child
Edited by Lena Rustin

Treating Phonological Disorders in Children. Metaphon - Theory to Practice
Janet Howell & Elizabeth Dean

Assessment and Management of Emotional and Psychosocial Reactions to Aphasia and Brain Damage
Peter Währborg

Group Encounters in Communication Disorders
Edited by Margaret Fawcus

Management of Acquired Aphasia in Children
Janet Lees

The Clinician's Guide to Linguistic Profiling of Language Impairment
Martin J Ball

Cluttering: A Clinical Perspective
Edited by Florence Myers & Kenneth O St Louis

Computers in Management and Therapy
Edited by David Rowley & Chris Code

Introductory Guide to Clinical Syntactic Analysis
Eeva Leinonen & Susan Fasler

Which Screen? A User's Guide to Speech and Language Screening Tests
Joanne Corcoran

Jumbly Words and Rights Where Wrongs Should Be

The Experience of Aphasia from the Inside

Edited By
Gill Edelman and Robert Greenwood

Far Communications
Kibworth

Copyright 1992 by **Far Communications Ltd.**, 5 Harcourt Estate, Kibworth, Leics. LE7 0NE, Great Britain.

All rights reserved.

No part of this book may be reproduced by any means, nor transmitted, nor translated into a machine language without the written permission of the publishers.

British Library Cataloguing in Publication Data:

Jumbly Words and Rights Where Wrongs Should Be:Experience of Aphasia from the Inside. - (Far Communication Disorders Series)
  I. Edelman, Gill II. Series
  616.85

ISBN 0-9514728-7-9

Cover by Artphics

Printed in England

Contents

Foreword   viii

Preface   ix

Introduction   1

CHAPTER 1   5

    Onset: "Something was very wrong."
    Marius Pope, Charles Edward Noden, Lily Reid, D.C. Wordley, J.E. Lyall

CHAPTER 2   15

    Realisation: "Then the enormity of the catastrophe that had befallen me seeped through my damaged brain."
    Mrs. Corner, Teresa Middleton, Danny, Leslie King, Licy Rosenberg, Mrs. E. Barber

CHAPTER 3   23

    Interactions: " ...if people would be more understanding ..."
    Anon (35 year old mother of two),,Anon (64 year old married woman), Mr. A.P., Mr.H., Anon, Monique, Malcolm G. Hampton, Male patient, Jack Hughes, Audrey Hope, Mary Mulqueen, Mrs. H., Jim.

CHAPTER 4   47

Adaptation: "A way of life changed in a minute of time."
Christine Bayliss, Anon (Speech Therapist), Betty Byers Brown (Speech Therapist), Daughter, Grand-daughter: Sarah White (Speech Therapist), Vera West, Ron Hudson, Robert Greenwood.

CHAPTER 5   73

Recovery: "I don't believe in the Resurrection ... but there is something going on up there!"
Terry Scott, Anon (19 year old girl), R.D. Thair, John Graney, Maria, Richard Bailey, Anon (wife of stroke patient), Mary Van Wyke, Susan Butler, Mr. D. Mott, Peter Heywood.

CHAPTER 6   103

The Future: "Has the brain reached the utmost of its healing? .... Ay, there's the rub."
Mr. B.M., M. Hopirott, John Hughes, Terry Dorsett, John, Laura, Tom (husband and wife), Arthur J. West, John Wells.

Proceeds from this book go to **Action for Dysphasic Adults (ADA)**. ADA was founded in 1980 by its current President Diana Law MBE., FCST (Hon), who is herself dysphasic. ADA is a registered Charity working to improve the quality of life of people with aphasia and their carers. It is the only organization in the United Kingdom with this purpose.

The aims of ADA are:

- providing information, advice and support to dysphasic people and their carers;

- increasing awareness and understanding of aphasia amongst healthcare professionals and the general public;

- funding research into aphasia and improved methods of treatment;

- campaigning for better therapy and support services for dysphasic people.

ADA needs support. You can contact ADA for information or to become a member at the following address:

> Action for Dysphasic Adults
> Canterbury House
> 1 Royal Street
> London SE1 7LN
> Tel: (071) 261 9572

FOREWORD

Dr Miriam Stoppard

Aphasia is a serious and complex communication disorder which can impair the ability to speak, read and write. It is caused by damage to the language centre of the brain following a stroke, head injury or brain disease.

Despite the fact that it affects 250,000 people in the United Kingdom, the condition is little known or understood. Following the onset of aphasia peoples' lives change. They have to come to terms with new situations, new roles and often changed relationships. Much of what we take for granted, listening to the radio, watching television, reading books, can be difficult for dysphasic people. They are cut off from all these avenues of communication and this often leaves people lonely and isolated.

Jumbly Words and Rights Where Wrongs Should Be: The Experience of Aphasia from the Inside has been written mostly by dysphasic people and gives a vivid insight into how they have come to terms with their condition, demonstrating the strength, courage and resilience of the human spirit. Aphasia reduces written and verbal skills but sufferers develop new and different ways to express themselves in response to this disability. **Jumbly Words** shows clearly that while aphasia may affect the way we communicate, intelligence and creativity are still intact.

PREFACE

Most books on the subject for the general public are written by doctors or by psychologists. The reason for this that both believe that because they have learnt a lot about the brain, they are qualified to write about dysphasic patients with the utmost confidence.

Speech therapists have also studied the brain and their day to day contact with dysphasic patients makes tham, I should think, more competent to understand the problems.

What about me, a retired lecturer in physical chemistry at a University? What do I know about the brain? Nothing at all. The reason I am involved in this book is because after a by-pass operation I had a severe attack of dysphasia. I now surprise many people by my almost complete recovery. When my speech therapist, Gill Edelman, asked me if I would like to cooperate with her on this book I readily agreed. Subsequently I did learn something about the brain by reading books and by attending sesssions of group therapy at City University, London. The people I met had all had a stroke and subsequent dysphasia. They varied considerably from those with small difficulties in speaking to those who had immense difficulty and who were not able to speak and had been in this position for up to five years. I enjoyed myself in these groups in a social way and because I was able to set an example for them to try and achieve. After a life time of physical chemistry, it was not easy by any means to write an account of the problems af dysphasia and particularly at the beginning when I was so very near to my own stroke.

I can understand the need for a book such as this because whenever I meet, read about or see on the television people with brain damage, I am with them. I am convinced that a book of this kind will be very useful to patients and their relatives as well as to doctors and I think it makes a very readable book for the general public.

Robert Greenwood

INTRODUCTION

Gill Edelman

Aphasia is a language disorder which affects approximately 250,000 people a year in the United Kingdom. It is caused by damage to the areas of the brain which control speech and language and can occur as the result of a stroke, head injury or other cerebral insult.

An individual who could previously communicate normally through both the spoken and written word may experience sudden devastation of these skills. Understanding of the spoken word, verbal expression, reading, writing and gesture may all be affected. The severity and pattern of the deficits varies according to the site and size of the area of damaged tissue in the brain. In severe cases, unable to understand what is said, to utter more than a few meaningless sounds, or to read or write, the individual may be locked into a private world where normal communication is impossible. At the other end of the scale, the individual with mild aphasia may experience only minor problems such as hesitancy in word-finding, or difficulty following a group discussion. Others may be totally unaware of these deficits. Between these extremes there is an enormous variety in the nature and extent of the disorder.

Patterns of recovery are equally varied and to some extent unpredictable. Some individuals may make a rapid and almost complete recovery, whilst others may make only very slow and painstaking progress over a considerable period of time. These individuals may have to live with their residual deficits and the restrictions these impose on their daily life.

It cannot be stressed enough that **no two aphasic patients are alike.** This is true, of course, not only in relation to the clinical symptoms but also in the way in which individuals react to the experience of aphasia. One of the reasons why recovery patterns are unpredictable, is that recovery depends not only on tangible factors such as the site and size of the lesion, the age of the individual and the quality of therapeutic intervention, but also on other factors such as the individual's personality, his level of motivation and the availability of emotional, psychological and social support.

It is difficult for us to imagine what it is like to be suddenly unable to understand or speak and to imagine how we would react to such a traumatic event. The irony is, of course, that the very fact of the communication handicap usually prevents individuals from expressing their feelings and sharing their experience.

This book has therefore been compiled in an attempt to reflect both the universal and individual experience of aphasia. Rather than writing a theoretical text we have asked the patients and their families, and indeed their speech therapists to speak for themselves. Through Speech Therapy Departments and the newsletter of Action for Dysphasic Adults (ADA) we requested contributions to a book about "What it is like to become aphasic ..... or to live with an aphasic partner ..... or to work with aphasic patients." The response was heartwarming.

Many of the contributors are looking back over their experience. For many of those with aphasia it may only be several years after the event that they have recovered sufficiently to put their experience into words. Others are still obviously struggling through the aphasia to express themselves. In editing this book we have tried to be as non-intrusive as possible. We have neither amended nor corrected any pieces sent to us. (We have, however, abbreviated some pieces which were too long to be reproduced in full and have removed any identifying names of hospitals, therapists, doctors, etc.)

Our task as editors then, was primarily to develop an overall framework for the book and to fit the pieces in to this framework in order to make a cohesive whole. The first chapter therefore, deals with the sudden onset of

THE EXPERIENCE OF APHASIA

aphasia and those which follow parallel the stages in recovery, until the final chapter which looks towards the future. We have refrained from any editorial comment throughout the book. There is no interlinking text; the pieces stand alone and speak for themselves. It would be wrong to suggest, however, that there is no editorial interpretation. We have carefully selected the pieces for each chapter and the order in which they should appear. The deliberate juxtaposition of particular pieces may serve to underline common strands of feeling or highlight contradictory reactions and responses.

The book contains an enormous mix of moods, both positive and negative. It is our sincere hope that as a whole, the book makes a balanced statement and that it will contribute to a deeper awareness and understanding of the experience of aphasia.

We would like to give our thanks to all the contributors for their commitment to this book, to Jacqueline Edelman who painstakingly typed every draft of the manuscript faithfully replicating every dysphasic spelling error, and finally all proof readers for whom this book presents an unforgettable challenge.

Chapter 1

ONSET

"Something was very wrong."

My Stroke

The 8.27 train to Cannon Street was already pulling into the platform when I arrived at Tunbridge Wells station that morning and because of this I hurried a bit and found a seat in the front end of the train. Usually when I'm on time I stroll down to the other end where there is usually more room.

However I found a seat and took my Telegraph out of my attache case. The case went on the rack. I unfolded the paper and started to read. The train moved and immediately I felt that something was very wrong.

I didn't feel in the slightest bit ill and I couldn't pinpoint it. But I felt that something, some "happening", something important had happened. Vaguely I thought that the happening was located in my face. I felt my cheek. It seemed OK. Moreover I could read without difficulty.

I decided that I was imagining it and I planned to go on to Cannon Street and the office. If anything had happened, I thought, I could always take the next train back.

By this time we had stopped at High Brooms and I thought: We'll stop once more at Tonbridge. Should I get off there?

But first I'd go and look at my face. If the jaw was slack of my face showed any other unusual sign I'd leave the train and telephone my wife to collect me.

I went to the lavatory. My face looked back at me in the mirror, refreshingly normal. I opened my mouth and closed it. All seemed OK. I tried to say "I feel quite well" and I couldn't make a sound except a moaning noise. It was frightening.

I returned to collect my coat and my case. I folded my newspaper and put my coat on. We were pulling into Tonbridge and I went to the door on the platform side.

There is a public telephone on the platform and it was occupied. After a while the man left it saying "It's out of order". I tried it and couldn't get a response, so I started walking from the station.

Next to the news kiosk in the entrance hall I saw another telephone. just outside the door a young man and a girl were locked in an embrace. I tapped them and moaned something and they let me pass.

I dialled home and Pat's reassuring voice answered. "Hello," she said, "Hello, who is it?"

"Hummbri ...." I bellowed "Hummbri, hummbri, hummbri ..."

She recognised my voice "Marius, is that you?" she said.

"Hummbri, hetmi ... hummbri hetmi." I bellowed back.

"Is it a joke? Is this a joke of some sort?" It was April 1.

"Hummbri, hummbri ... hetmi, hetmi, hummbri ...."

Suddenly her voice was precise, cool. "I understand," she said. "You're in Tonbridge. I'm coming to get you. Don't move from the station." And she repeated: "I'm coming to get you. Don't move from the station."

I put down the phone and walked outside. It was raining, but I didn't care. I walked up the road and stood outside the Safeway store, watching the shoppers.

I thought I'm finished. It's my last day or two. It'll all be over soon. I was surprised that I felt calm about it.

THE EXPERIENCE OF APHASIA

A little later I noticed that there was a lot of traffic in this part of the main road. Mostly because I didn't want a delay before I was taken to hospital I decided to walk up the hill and stand where she'd see me and could turn the car easily. I walked as far as Brook Street and waited in the rain.

She saw me immediately and turned into the island to pick me up. Patrick was with her, looking anxious.

"I'll take you home and phone the doctor right away" she said.

I wanted to go to hospital. "Otal, otal" I said.

"No, it'll be better at home. The doctor will come soon."

She was right. A doctor arrived within ten minutes. I didn't know him. He asked me questions, some of them seemingly idiotic.

"What's this?" he asked, pointing to his tie. "Hi". "And this?" "Hen". (It was his pen). "And this?" "Hirt" (shirt).

I picked up a pen and paper and wrote: "I haven't lost my marbles, you know, only my voice."

He was not in the least affronted. Patiently he explained to me what I had already guessed - that he suspected that I'd had a slight stroke and that he was attempting to discover what part of the brain it affected.

He said that in the majority of these cases speech began to return to the patient within a relatively short time and that he'd be back in the evening to see how much progress I'd made.

After he left I tried to talk. I felt very light hearted. The whole thing had changed into a huge joke and I exploited this mostly to assuage the worries of Patrick who was showing signs of alarm.

My efforts became more and more comic and we all ended up convulsed in laughter. The joke of the day became my efforts to say "double-adaptor" when I asked for such a device so that I could have both a radio and a lamp next to my armchair.

The doctor returned in the evening and decided that I hadn't made much progress and that I would be better off in hospital.

I arrived at the hospital in an ambulance feeling a total fraud. Apart from a speech defect, I felt as well as at any time during the past few years.

That night I lay in bed surrounded by men who where really ill and whose hearts were being monitored. It was an unexpected end to a day which had started so happily.

Marius Pope
Written early 1983

Had a stroke 21 Sept 1987 --- One week before, I was at work and I lost the use of my **left arm** for about five minutes. I went to see my doctor as my wife thought I'd had a slight stroke. He said it was arthritus - I continued working all the next week and seemed be unable to walk completely straight - something seemed to be causing me to keep going over a little to the right. (After I'd had the stroke my workmates said they had noticed this.)

On the morning of the 21st Sep I went to work on the 6 am till 2 pm shift. I didn't feel too well and the problem of walking straight seemed to worsten.

I came home at 2 pm. Had a good dinner and felt much better. I decided later to paint the shed door - I did about half of this and all of a sudden I had a terrible pain across my stomach and I lost the use of my **right arm**. I managed to walk into the house my wife told me later I was dragging my right leg. I didn't realize I could not speak until my wife asked me what was wrong. She also said my face was very distorted. I remember

THE EXPERIENCE OF APHASIA

being taken to the hospital in the ambulance - having my heart tested and all the doctors asking me what had happened but I could not answer them. I don't remember being taken to the ward. I remember being so very tired and wishing they would let me go to sleep.

The men on the ward were talking to me. I understood what they were saying but I could not answer them - the words would not come out.

When I went for speach therapy I could not understand what she was talking about it meant nothing to me. The objects she had meant nothing to me. I could not recognize them at all.

I seemed to lose all track of time - but I could walk. I could not understand why I could not hold a spoon or fork - I could not find my mouth sometimes. The nurses kept telling me "You'll be alright Eddie don't worry". I was taken for a scan - I didn't know where I was going but the journey made me terribly sick. The ambulance man cleaned me up.

I was very frightened when they were doing the scan I wondered what was happening and why they had fastened me down. I felt very emotional and cried a lot something I have never done before.

When I came back from having the scan I was told I could go home - I didn't want to as I felt so ill.

After I got home I was still feeling so very tired. I could not bath myself as I felt so weak so my wife used to bath me. I still could not talk very much. I was very frustrated when people could not understand me. I would sit and look at pictures - I knew what some of them were but others I had no idea what they were. I could not remember names even those of my children and grandchildren. My speach therapist gave me tests to do - at first I found them very hard but gradually with her help and the help of my family things got a lot better.

When I first started to remember things I could not sleep at night there seemed to be so much going on in my head. I would try to remember my

JUMBLY WORDS

doctors name - I couldn't and it would bother me so much I had to waken my wife and ask her. She would say Dr.____ and I would say it over and over again - but when I woke up the next morning I still had no idea what his name was it was as if my brain would not work. I think that is the worse thing about a stroke not being able to remember. My wife would give me clues - even the first letter of a word - but it meant nothing to me.

Now four months later I still forget things and when I am tired my speach is not very good. I can do my tests from my speach therapist but I need a lot of time to do them. Words still seem to get mixed up. If I walk too far I am still very tired. I don't feel at all like I used to do. I have no energy. I was a very active man before I had this stroke.

I get a lot of pain in my right arm whether this is from the stroke or due to arthritus I don't know. My arm has lost all its strenght and I dont have much grip in it. I wish there had been some therapy I could have had for it but I was told it was not needed. I used a hard ball and a soft ball of my own to try to get the grip back. I know I have been one of the lucky ones, but I wish it had never happened to me and I could me as fit and strong as I was before.

Charles Edward Noden
January 1987

I remember feeling ill and telling my husband that I would not get up this morning, and would he telephone the Doctor at 9 a.m.

I had noticed a kind of numbness in my right hand during the preceding days, felt very tense and worried. It was four in the afternoon when the Doctor came, and by this time my husband had sent for my daughter and son-in-law and also for my son who lives in Majorca.

THE EXPERIENCE OF APHASIA

On the way to the hospital I was totally confused and could not understand what was happening to me. The medical staff, Doctors and Nurses were so kind and caring - I could feel this through my confusion and fears - they were doing all they could to help me.

When the examinations were completed and my husband and family were told that I had suffered a stroke, I was put into bed. One thought hammered into my brain - I knew that my daughter and her family were going to Majorca on holiday within a few days and I wanted to tell her not to postpone it, but I could not speak a word. However, she knew what was on my mind. Eventually, my family went home and I was made comfortable for the night. The last thing my nurse did for me was to lift up the rails of my bed so that I would not fall out.

Then the enormity of the catastrophy that had befallen me seeped through my damaged brain. I had the most awful headache, my right arm was paralysed and I was rendered speechless. The loneliness and devastation I felt within me was soul destroying. Being unable to communicate with other people, and losing memory for simple words - words like "drink of water", "toothbrush", "open", "shut" and the like.

I was told by my nurse one morning to see if I could wash and dress myself. I was willing to do this, but oh the time it took me to wash. Getting dressed was a nightmare! The domestic lady came whilst I was struggling and in tears and she lent a helping hand.

The first words I was able to speak were addressed to a young lady who was accompanying the lady Doctor who was doing the rounds of the ward. Her dress was so pretty, mauve, lilac and blue, and without thinking, I said "I like your dress". The Doctor was most surprised and so was the wearer of the dress!

A social worker came to visit me whilst I was in hospital and she asked me questions as to what kind of a house I lived in, did I have a husband,

JUMBLY WORDS

how did I think I would cope etc. etc.

When she left me, I began to take stock of myself and circumstances, and from that moment onwards I resolved not to become a cabbage. To communicate, to become interested in what went on around me, laugh at my mistakes. To learn to write with my left hand and to exercise my right hand. To get out in the kitchen, to learn again how to make a cake, a Yorkshire pudding and above all, to keep my keen sense of humour.

It still takes me ages to write a letter, the words are in my head, but I have great difficulty in transferring them to paper.

I cannot add up or take-away, but I think I speak quite well, providing I do not keep on too long!

I try to count my blessings and believe that I have been very lucky.

Lily Reid
December 1986

My mind sits on the fence
It is cocooned with cotton wool;
Impervious to worry.
I live outside myself,
Free from the useless limbs.
I can hear everything -
But I cannot speak!
I have warmth and benevolence -
I stay on my fence,
Isolated.

THE EXPERIENCE OF APHASIA

I sit unshaven in my chair,
Boring, discomfort skirts my
Unending echo, touching my
Feelings with memory, vaguely,
Tells me something!!
I cannot tell the nurse
My name is ? ? ?

The tea, the coffee breaks the day,
The temperature, the blood pressure.
Unwanting help, hidden in myself,
I see my friends and family -
I know them, - I need them!
But I can tell them nothing,
Whilst moisture flecks my eye
And wets the mouth,
Unspeaking.

Now I know some patient, friends,
Cheerful, helpful nurses smile warmly.
I feel tired by 8.00
I have a warm, drowziness,
At nine Sister sees me comfortable,
A kind "Goodnight" leaves me
In an embryonic curl,
Eyes shut, I feel warmth
and - belonging.

JUMBLY WORDS

I hear disembodied voices,
The noises round the ward,
I try to think, but thoughts
Are locked away.
I cannot say a prayer -
Just "Our Father" nothing else -
"Our Father", - allows me -
A Peaceful Sleep!!!

D.C. Wordley
Written on January 15th., 1979 (20 months after a stroke).

One does not raely rember having a stoke. All you kown is lying in bed with people coming and going.

Time means nothing to you, is didnt to me bacause I could not tell the time. Enwt I realiesd that there was someing wrong with my leg and my right hand. It dawed on me evenaly that I was slighly pasilised. But woset was to come I couldt spekeng very well I could not make Im sefl unertood. The dortors must have todold me that I had a stoke. It was nice to be taken to X ray, speak therapy, to see other pealopie that made the day shorter. Visitors were nice to get allthough you coudle not speke very well.

That is why speke therapy is very imompet to me.

It is a year since I had the stoke my pogesrs is very good. But things are very vague as what is was like to have a stoke.

J. E. Lyall

Chapter 2

REALISATION, PROBLEMS, REACTIONS

"Then the enormity of the catastrophe that had
befallen me seeped through my damaged brain."

In this last year I have found out a great deal about speech. It is far more complicated than I ever knew.

In the beginning, I thought that once I could make sounds and then words, I would be "home and dry".

After some months I found that, at times, names would elude me, but I could remember the first letter of the names. After a few minutes of probing around I would remember the whole name.

I lost my speech 25.9.85. Since then, when I forget a name, no longer does the first letter comes to mind; after a pause the whole emerges.

Often, these are names of people that I'd almost forgotten.

Mrs. Corner
October 1986

    Semi-skilled milk.
    Hamshit.
    Jumbley words and wrongs where rights should be.

JUMBLY WORDS

Gaps where words should be. And wrongs tensed.
Senses back to front and puzzles expressions
trying to understand my thoughts ... thoughts
clear as bells but come out so muffled and jangled.
Yes for nos and whole nos have gone.
And whole words die and
Friends say it doesn't matter.
It matters for me. The frustration is intense
and painful and makes me feel so mad and crazy.
Its getting worse and its here in black and white.
Jumbly, sometimes giggly ...
squeen of hearts. And new words form ... lazy words
marry eachother and the gaps goone.
Lots of examples I've forgotten now ... memory
gone and paerhaps thats why the gaps come andgo.
Feel that practise makes perfect. Word perfect.
Try hard to keep it sane, to speak to you but
is it in vain? Can't accept that its really me.
Someone else doing the wrong bits.
I've always written so weel ... Spoken so well.
Why not now? Called you him and her me and
and them those ... it gets worse and I rty to
keep it ... try to carry on speaking to you.

Teresa Middleton
May 1987

THE EXPERIENCE OF APHASIA

I was at work when I lost my voice I was couldt with work and when sat done I was caught A and D who saud U gad a stroke.

I was on the 5th floor for 5 days it caught evan yes and no I got a patient for shave me as lost the use on the arm and my face drop and I kept dropping.

The "doctor" was I got home and attend speech tharapist here. I was introduced to her who taught me thumb up was yes and "no" then I came a good news lesson which "oo" and "ah" I was terrified, my people could'nt understand me, my wife couldnt give at enough help I understand other people my arm got better and the face on normal.

I am speech therapist and got yes and no the two weeks and I learned whith the first help with wife and Catherine they taught and help and I could get bye. I get lonely at times and want to cried and nots so much now.

I get up to the speech therapist at 8.30 daily and I take noticed and learn at home.

Danny
Aged 63 years.

My first personal experience of dysphasia was really extraordinary. I was already charibound for 9 yrs, with cerebral atrophy, but had accepted that, and then in May 1986, I was on holiday with my wife at a disabled holiday home, at Bursledon near Southampton and really enjoying myself. On the final evening, there was plenty of laughing and joking with friends we had made during our stay there. Went to bed very happy, had a good nights sleep but on waking next morning, I could not speak, I thought I had strained my throat laughing too much. On arriving home, my wife called in the Doctor, and straight away she said I had had a slight stroke, which affected my speech. I was dumbfounded. The Doctor then arranged for a speech therapist to visit me, and I had no idea what to expect. But I was soon to find out. When the therapist arrived, a very pleasant lady, she asessed me, to find out what affects the stroke had had on me, speechwise. She comes every week, and gets me to pronounce certain words and sounds, what at the time made me feel like a child again, but now I know the object of the exercise. Very interesting. The words I found most difficult, were those beginning - S-T, but have now conquered that. Now it is - SQU - SKW - but with practise, it is slowly coming back. Now my advice to fellow patients is, never give up - cooperate with your therapist, and you will win in the end.

Leslie King

I think it was a Monday norming and I think my friend was worried. Everything was very hazy for me. My friend rang the doctor and the doctor came at elevenish. I remember that she said it would be good to go to the hospital. But I don't remember how. I was in bed. The next time I remember I was in bed in the hospital.

There were some nurses and they were talking, - something connected with me. I didn't understand everything. They talked to each other and I was annoyed because I couldn't speak. I was so annoyed and frustrated. I couldn't speak. When I think about it I still feel frustrated.

Facing my bed people were coming in and out of the doors. On the

THE EXPERIENCE OF APHASIA

doors there was a design in black and white like flowers. It didn't bother me, it was neither pleasing nor aggravating. I think I was there three weeks, and somebody must have said that I said something about the design, and they told me it was printed "close the door". I suppose I realised they were letters but I was indifferent.

The speech therapist was a great help and very patient - a lovely man. He came a few times in the afternoon. He had some pictures, and printed words with only three letters. And this started to make some sense. Things became clearer. I still remember the pictures! But I don't remember what my speech was like when I left the hospital.

Occasionally two or three times in the morning they collected me with the ambulance and I went to the hospital to see the speech therapist. It was a nuisance, I liked to be there, I saw him for only half an hour but I had to be there the whole morning. They collected me at half past eight and brought me home at luch time. I couldn't read of course. Sometimes I thought I'm not going, its boring. But it was good to have the speech therapy. I always wanted to get on with it. Then I didn't go anymore.

My friends took me for walks and came to see me a lot. One friend helped with making me write and read and doing figures. I didn't realise how terrible my speech must have been. Eventually one friend tried to contact a speech therapist - but this therapist only worked with children, but she recommended somebody else to come to the house.

I realised by then I needed help and I was very happy to have help but I still felt indifferent about my speech. In a way I had given up. One is detached.

When I knew I would get some help I began to be involved to talk. The thoughts were there but they do not come out - no sound! I always was looking forward to see the speech therapist.

In my nature I always wanted to get on. Even now I wanted to get out on my own.

Now I can talk but I still can't spell. I have to use a dictionary a lot. The easiest words I can't spell, but of course other people don't know I can't spell. I know I will never be alright. My age is against me as well. Sometimes I didn't realise the words are wrong. Even though I am not English I have the feeling for the language, and that I was wrong. Other people didn't comment, but I'm sure they knew it.

Now I have books from the library with large print only, the ones that interest me. I read aloud even in bed on my own, otherwise it doesn't sink in. If the author writes interesting things and with an easy style I can grasp it. Sometimes I have to go over and over again because it doesn't sink in. If I get tired I have to stop in the middle as it doesn't get in that brain!

I got the prepositions and pronouns, more than he's and she's, wrong. I didn't always know it either. My speech therapist helped tremendously and with getting my books. Reading helps of course, because it makes me more fluent. I remember words more easily when I talk. I realise only now that I don't have a problem with prepositions and pronouns.

I get rusty if I don't talk to people, especially face-to-face. If there is a third person I shut up as I am not quick enough to respond. I like to have people visit me at home, just one at a time, then I have the benefit of their speech.

While I was in hospital I didn't feel myself - there was somebody else in my skin. And for some months afterwards my friends helped me to find myself, and today I feel myself again.

Licy Rosenberg
February 1987

THE EXPERIENCE OF APHASIA

I had a small stroke in April 1983, and another one in December 31st to begin with it, I couldn't speak and I couldn't recognise anything, my brain was nothing. My daughter took me home for 15 weeks, a month a I didn't remember, I started in February with a therapist at Brighton Hospital. I started reading, on a paper 2 or 3 words, then my daughter helped me, doing words writing and reading, some days I'd cry but went back again.

Then on April, I went home. I hated it, but you must help yourself, 4, 5, 6, 7 8 and 9 months, then I went on my own to Norfolk, went on a bus to London then changed to Norfolk, I was there with a friend for 2 weeks, I felt very good talking, reading and especially writing. I went to hospital in November with my therapist she was a brilliant person especially for me, I'm nearly better, the time will come and I'll be hundred per cent, but I've finished with the therapist.

Thank you all.

Mrs. E. Barber

Chapter 3

INTERACTIONS

"....if people would be more understanding."

Used to be terrible when I first had the stroke and I were talking to that old lady in Ward 4 and I couldn't tell her that I couldn't tell my name. She thought I were foreign "you not English are you?"
    There were another lady in Vic and I couldn't talk right. I lost some of it because I had a kidney infection and it knocked me back a bit and I couldn't remember nurses to tell about bedpans and things and then I wanted to phone Mick. I had it in my mind but I couldn't say when I wanted to on the phone and the lady opposite came to me and she said "What do you want?" and I had to explain to her that I wanted towels. Very very embarrassing.
    Just before I left hospital I was crying all day because I couldn't talk to anybody and I couldn't understand from anybody. I was just sitting there and then Christine came in .... but I couldn't tell her nowt.

Written by a 35 year old mother of two.

It's a year and three months since I had my stroke. My speech is much better now but sometimes words come forward and I'm going to speak and it goes back. I can say a thing but I can't say it quite right, I can think it

JUMBLY WORDS

and I can't say it, and my memory ...... it comes and goes. I give up sometimes and it makes me feel sad.

I feel frustrated and subdued. When people walk about me they all seem to have something going for them - it makes me feel queer, I feel I'm on my own a little ..... they don't know that I'm different. I don't go out much and I used to go out every day. I only go out when Brian or Sharon (My son and daughter) take me. I don't want to go out. I used to always be cheerful and I'm not now. My son says I never smile, I don't feel like smiling.

I always feel better when there's .... in the group, and there's all stroke victims. The group's enjoyable I always look forward to coming ..... we help one another with the work, it's very helpful.

Written by a 64 year old married woman.

It was a curious feeling of tiredness - there and then gone - that should have warned me but it didn't and so when it came the shock was all the greater.....

It happened on a Sunday lunch-time when the bottom fell out of my world so to speak and I ended up in hospital ten miles away. Unable to speak and unable to make myself understood despite being absolutely clear in my mind what I wanted to say. I can always remember one character in particular. He asked me a question I couldn't answer and there-after he didn't look at me. It was as if I wasn't there. He was still there when I left.

But he was talking and I was not. Very difficult. But I am gradually getting better. I feel much better in certain company than others. In some

THE EXPERIENCE OF APHASIA

cases I go utterly voiceless and the more I try the more difficult it gets and eventually I have to give up entirely. And yet, with others I can more or less chat away almost like normal.

Mr. A.P.,
Journalist.

One morning I woke and thought that I was alright, my wife and son were in their beds and so there was no-one to talk with. I walked down to town to sign on the dole as I was not working. I couldn't sign and I couldn't talk. So I went home. Later my wife said to me "Aren't you talking to me?" and I couldn't. The next day my brother-in-law came to the house and he was talking to me but I couldn't talk. I think that he went to his house and that my sister 'phoned a doctor about me. He came that night and he didn't know what was wrong with me. The next day another doctor came and this doctor sent me to the "nut house"... the people were okay and one Sister was the one who made me talk again. She said that if I wanted a match she would give it if I said "match". I couldn't say "match" but I said "yes". It was like an old rusty engine was turning on again and it nearly killed me to talk. For three or four days I couldn't do anything.

After a week and a day, they sent me to a hospital the north where I had a scan and a doctor told me I'd had a stroke. After the scan I was sent to another hospital where I stayed a week. My blood changed again and the doctor said that I could go home.

In Ward 10 of the hospital, it was large and, I think, that everyone who came to my bed gave me a blood test - even the cleaner!

When I came out everybody would talk to me for a small time and then walk off.

I can read a small while and then I forget what I was reading.

In my club I like snooker and sometimes some of my mates give me a game. I could play cards but I don't like them so I sit and look at the T.V.

I can't read a book because it takes too long.

If I go into a shop I can't talk to the shopkeeper and I can't hear the prices of the things I want.

If two or three people are talking I can't hear what they're talking about.

If I go into a pub, I don't know the price of a drink if someone says it. I have to see the price.

In my house, I sit down and watch the T.V. or listen to the radio. If I have a book I can try and read it, but if I read a while I forget or throw the book down.

Mr. H. 52 years old
2 years after his stroke.

(Mr. H. had a stroke which affected his speech, but there was no limb paralysis. He was admitted to the local psychiatric hospital until the correct diagnosis was made.)

I was ill.

Some people shout at me and I have to tell them that I did not have to shout. A fear of children very shortly gave me a head aches.

I still cannot say if value is suitable.

I used to try to make a cup of tea etc., put I could not understand what was so difficulty to consentrate.

THE EXPERIENCE OF APHASIA

I could not say if it was right or left.

In the shops I would forget what I wanted.

Men do not seem to be helpful.

I went for a walk I used to tell people that I was sorry that I didn't know places (I knew but I could not sa).

One day a woman who was taking the dog for a walk, she asked me about the flowers and I had to say that I had been ill the woman ran away as if I was a danger.

My right eye was slowly getting better and the Doctor told me to go to the Eye Infirmary. My wife had been with me and I was waiting then I was called.

I told the elderly Sister that I had been ill and could not speak very well.

I thought that I should have to go into another room and she said I was in the wrong room and I should see number three.

When I was asked for different letters I knew that I could not say which was right or wrong.

The first girl gave me back to the Sister and she told me which is her left.

I was very glad when I was taken into the correct waiting room.

Several of the other people who had been watching had to help.

She had made me feel so stupid although I had tried so hard to help.

Anon.

JUMBLY WORDS

I am 16 and I have had to change my life. Not being able to read, write or talk is no joke, and this is what happend about hafe a year ago.

I woke up in hospital. Some time later I tride to read a book but I was unable to understand. I was very shockt. What made it worse was that I was unable to see propally. But the worse thing was that people woude tell my that I was about to read and write and that I was not really triing hard enarf. If people would be more understanding and less pushy, but I can not expest people to understand I've they have never had a stroke.

Monique
December 1986

Frustration

A sit in hospital and session of pysiotherapy. I can see the good progress in variety patient to from for example wheelchair to walk themselves or to wash and dress themselves. It is help to strive to in improve themselves and in the patient in this hospital. It encourage the patients with touch of envy sometimes!

Feelings

List depression and frustration it worst feeling and helplessness.

THE EXPERIENCE OF APHASIA

Fear

Fear that I might cripple in the left am never again
Fear it again another stroke
Fear that the wife get ill again, such is rush in hospital/in summer 1986 to operation for appendicitis.

Work

I retire is a chartered building surveyor and can be never work again necessitated is 100% cure is a cannot climb ladder etc. is dictated wrote the concise report. Lack of confidence gradually improve. The my deputy suveyors to discuss from details. Some accounts. Encourage friends to visit and the grandchildren. Discuss work. Talk of the telephone and sit one committee.

Injury

Fear of another fall caused injury - in summer fell in the garden resulting in fractured wrist in plaster of 6 weeks also in sprain ankle. One stroke patient falls outside 3 times and one stroke patient has another stroke.

Inactive

Many frustrations is wife and helplessness and depression from not able to odd simple job can't do.

JUMBLY WORDS

Frustration

Because wife marvellous cover all financial, taxes, transport, foods etc. and organise move it new bungalow and continue to work.

    A good idea in sit in hospital and in session of pysiotherapy I can see the good progress in variety stroke patient from a wheelchair to walk themselves to wash and dress themselves. It help to discuss in progress in the patient in coffee break.

Malcolm G. Hampton

When I had my stroke, I felt very ill. The Doctor Came. he wanted me to go in Hospital, which I Refused.
    I had to have my Bed Downstairs Because I Could not go Upstairs
    My Cousins Looked after me.
    Washing me & Etc.
    After a Month The Lady Therapist
    They gave me all the Exercise
    Which went well.
    After a month they Discharge me.
    They were very Good
    Next came the Speech Therapist. My Speech was better for all Lessons she gave me. She comes Every Week or once a fortnight.
    She is very Good.
    I not using the Frame anymore.

THE EXPERIENCE OF APHASIA

I am going upstairs to my Room.

I go about around the House doing odd jobs. Like washing up & vacuum.

I can Shave my Self and Work.

I do not go out Walking a Lot but I go some places By Car.

But My Leg and Hand is not ready yet.

Man Aged 82
First stroke August 1986

Most people realize that no two persons have the same fingerprints. I would like to emphasize that it is the same thing with strokes: each one is different. Some leave the person disabled - arm or leg, both, at one side or the other - any part of the body can be affected. The speech, the thinking ability, reason, and the memory can be attacked.

I mention this because the matter I am going to discuss does not affect everybody who has a stroke, but the ones who have had similar problems to myself.

My stroke happened about 5 years ago and though it did not leave any physical defects on the body, it left me with dysphasia. Speech, thought, memory and concentration are all affected.

Most people think its only the speech that's affected; they do not see the effort it takes to remember the words (sometimes they don't come) and the thinking that's needed to construct them in a sensible way. People who know me better see this further handicap, but even the persons who are close me cannot see, before all the handicaps I have mentioned, is one of

JUMBLY WORDS

confidence.

Confidence is the one thing that is omitted when they list the handicaps caused by strokes. Speech, thinking, memory, etc. are all affected by this lack of confidence when you are face to face with someone. Once you are "on the spot", the concentration disappears and you are left devoid of any thoughts. Being on the phone is a classic example.

There are several parallels I could give in "real life". Take the person who for the first time is suddenly thrust into the glare of TV cameras, or the amateur actor who has "stage fright" and "dries up", or the little boy when asked to take a message by the headmaster, can't remember a word.

It is all too apparant to me when asked asked a question out of the blue, when faced with the simplest of calculation or even when you are asked how you are keeping, the mind, too often, is blank. The term I use for this is "emotionally stupid" or "the stupidity of embarrassment". I have it almost totally and Terry Wogan is at the other end of the scale!

The problem, basically, is one of confidence. How does one combat it? One way is by facing the problem; do not be afraid of being taken for a fool. Alternatively, you practice in your mind the words you most often need. One way is by writing. By writing you remove the "face to face" problem. You have all the time in the world to think of the words needed. Nobody is waiting, therefore one is not embarrassed and the stupidity does not arise. If the words appear my memory has won, if the words do not apear then my memory has lost - but it has been a fair struggle! I am not playing against loaded dice. I just sit down with a pen, paper and Roget's Thesaurus and the exercise does me good! It's a long, hard job, but it has its benefits.

Jack Hughes
(Written February 1987)

THE EXPERIENCE OF APHASIA

Mrs. Hope was eighty one when she had a stroke at the beginning of January 1986. She has a pacemaker and lives with her husband in a bungalow. In December 1986 she agreed to talk about how stroke affected her life, hoping that her experiences would encourage others who are dealing with stroke either in their own lives or their family, friends and neighbours.

Speech Therapist: What was it like when you came out of hospital and came back to live at home?
Mrs. Hope: It was nice to be home but I didn't understand what people were saying. When anyone came to talk to me I thought I talked different and didn't answer them. What does George think?
Mr. Hope: Well, she was a bit slow at speaking. She didn't speak for a few days.
Mrs. Hope: I didn't speak. I couldn't speak. When anyone came I was frightened to speak. It was terrible, terrible. I was glad to be home, you know, but it was awful.
Speech Therapist: What was the worst bit?
Mrs. Hope: Well, not being able to speak was the worst.
Speech Therapist: You didn't have any words at all.
Mrs. Hope: No, no words at all. Then it came back gradually, mind I helped it come back. I talked to George, you know, and I talked to the family but when anybody else came in I was dead you know.
Speech Therapist: So you made an effort with people you knew.
Mr. Hope: Especially some people. She can speak to some people better than others.
Mrs. Hope: I can talk to you ordinary. I can answer the 'phone. But some people that come to the door, I'm always dithering, can't answer them, no. I get upset you know.

Speech Therapist: Have you any thoughts on this?

Mr. Hope: Well, I think perhaps when she's feeling a bit tired she, you get confused at times.

Mrs. Hope: When I'm tired I don't know what's what. When I'm not tired I'm fine. If a knock comes to the door I go to answer it but I have to have him behind me because I don't know what to say. Like the pop man came today so I got my purse and rushed to the door like I would have but when he came I didn't know what to say.

Speech Therapist: What did you want to say?

Mrs. Hope: I wanted to give him two bottles and get three but he hesitated when I gave him the two bottles and I said "I want three". Then George came of course and everything's all right when he's there.

Speech Therapist: Do you find it easier to talk when George is there?

Mrs. Hope: Oh yes, yes. I find it awful strange to talk when he's not.

Speech Therapist: So its like having some moral support.

Mrs. Hope: Yes, that's right.

Writing

Mrs. Hope had been a prolific letter writer before her stroke, in fact she had been George's pen pal before they had met and married. Immediately after her stroke she found she could not write, but soon was able to write the names of shopping items. Gradually her ability to write sentences returned. Here she describes some of the difficulties she faced.

Mrs. Hope: Every word I'm going to write I can spell but when I come to write it I write it upside down, like 'i' before 'e', yet I can spell every word.

Mr. Hope: It doesn't come out right. I can tell you that.

THE EXPERIENCE OF APHASIA

Speech Therapist: Yes, you know what letters you want to write.

Mrs. Hope: Oh yes I know what letters I want to write and I get my paper and I'm writing and when I read it its all funny.

Speech Therapist: Yes, you've always been able to spot your spelling errors haven't you.

Mrs. Hope: So, I had to write slow to get my spelling right you know.

Speech Therapist: Yes. I remember when you were trying to spell George.

Mrs. Hope: Yes. G-o-r-g-e. I spelt it like that for ages, but I can get it now. All the names I can spell, Diane, Don, Alison, and Karen, and June and Tony, I can spell them all.

Speech Therapist: How did you get on with the Christmas cards this year?

Mrs. Hope: Oh, I write them funny. I can write "From George and Audrey" but I cannot put any greetings, you know. He addresses the envelopes.

Recalling Names

Mr. Hope: She gets very mixed up with names, like our grand-daughters Alison and Karen. You often mix them up, don't you? She says Alison instead of Karen and Diane instead of Ann.

Mrs. Hope: The little girl that lives over there, she's lived over there about sixteen years and I do know her name, "Erren", but if she's coming out there I would never think of it.

Speech Therapist: Have you made any changes since you had your stroke?

Mrs. Hope: Well, no. You see I'm one of these people that must be on the go. I cannot rest so I cannot change. He thinks I should make changes. He thinks I should sit here and talk but I cannot sit here and talk and talk.

JUMBLY WORDS

Speech Therapist: So what do you do?

Mrs. Hope: Move the furniture round.

Speech Therapist: Have you moved all this furniture round on your own?

Mrs. Hope: I moved that from there. It took me ages and ages but I did it. Every time he escape I usually push, then sit down, you know. But Donald brought the table down and of course we have a home help and I do more for her coming than when she doesn't come.

Speech Therapist: You mean you get it tidy.

Mrs. Hope: I get up and I wash up and wash the things and do all kinds before she comes. And he says "You're daft you know" but I must have it right.

A final thought for those who like to help.

Mrs. Hope describes her feelings soon after she had returned home from hospital.

"I could've told them I'd never go out again because everyone looked at you. When I'm out, if I drop anything people are always fussing to pick it up where they wouldn't have before I had the stroke. Then I thought - Heavens, they must know I'm bad."

The following piece was written by Mrs. Hope.

Well about a year ago I was in hospital with a bad heart attack. I have had pacemaker for nine years, (the first pacemaker of that type that was done in Britain from America) that was almost for years ago, however I got home for Christmas, which was very good, but I was not very well. Then one Saturday evening I just fell to the floor, I knew nothing else. My husband sent for the doctor, I had had a stroke. I woke up in hospital with my family sitting round me. I did not know what had happened. I could not talk, not understand. When they went away I felt lost and lonley.

THE EXPERIENCE OF APHASIA

nobody spoke to me except the nurses and I did not know what they were saying I could not swallow and eat or drink it was all on my lelt side and my right temple ached, also I had pain in my right side. I just laid quiet, (I think so) I was in a corner and just watched. Then they sent a speech therinist (a Miss -) she was wonderfull, I did not understand her, but she gave me hope. she arranged to come when my grandchildren were there and she asked them to bring some photos, they did that and I was able to tell her, in my round about way who they were, she seemed to spend **hours** with me, (that hours would just be minuits) but I used to watch for her coming she was wonderfull. When I came home, after a while I got Speech Theratist from here, she is Mrs. -, she is lovely, (all the Speech Thirpist must be lovely). she has learned me very good, she likes my home work and has learned me all she can (so she said), but I can learn lots from her. I have had quite a lot of hospital from her, I had a fall down the steps, and was five weeks in hospital I came out walking ons ticks, but I feel better now, but my husband cannot leave me. I fall down and when I get down I cannot get up, it is awful he cannot leave me, but a car comes to pick me up, so I get carryed with thise other persons to the clinic, it is good, six of us, some cannot speak, two of us can talk, but the ones that cannot speak have lots of qualities that I have not got, they can count and reckoning comes easy, it does not with me, my mind seems blank, although I can spell the words, I still wright worng, please excuse the mistakes, my husband was in the merchant navy and I wrote to him every **days** for years so you can tell what writing meant to me. I **can** wright, but lots of things the others can do, **I cannot**.

Audrey Hope
December 6th 1986

JUMBLY WORDS

On Friday the 5th November 1982 I was at work waiting for the day to finish as my husband Jim and I were going on the Monday to Majorca for a week's break before Christmas.

Around 10 o'clock that morning I became unwell and Jim was called for. He brought me home and called the doctor. After she examined me she sent me to the hospital and it was there it was discovered that I had suffered a slight stroke and in doing so I lost my speech and the use of my right arm. During the next few weeks I was in hospital I was crying when my family and my friends came to visit me. I thought I would never speak again and was worried about what people would think of me. With the hospital care and attention in a couple of months the use of my right hand returned. Although weak and still is, I can use it.

My speech is slowly returning. I attend Speech Therapy on Wednesday at the hospital and on a Friday there is group therapy.

Being cheerful has helped me an awful lot of the way. Going out to the shops helps me to become independant. When I go out, if I tell people I had a stroke they are nice to me and have more time for me. Sometimes I get hot and bothered if someone upsets me and the words don't come out.

Keep going and you'll get there in the long run.

Mary Mulqueen

THE EXPERIENCE OF APHASIA

At 21st May I woke up with a bad dream. I dont usually by troubled by such things and I felt quite well. I decided to get up and make some tea. I was just over recovering had a double hip replancent so I was a little slow, so that by the time was the tea ready I was expecting my home helf, and when I heard her key in her lock I called out "Tea up" (or something of the sort). This is not difficult to say but I could produce something that even I see was nonsense. I tried again - with the result. I seemed to have become an idiot. Luckly my home helf had some experence of strokes and asked me who was my doctor. I could find my diary and she rang her and touther and with a very good friend they got me to the hospital.

I was absolute terrfied. I had heard of strokes but had thought they usually died of them. In fact I hoped this one would, and as and the quicker the better. I didn't realise that they could be treated.

Next Mornday I realised I could read a few a letters, but only single words - no sencenes. Speaking was in the roughyng the position. I seemed to be in the Geriatric ward which was not encouring. The first I thing saw was a large clock. I knew what it was for but it had no message for me at all. I supposed was that due shock but this turned out one of one most diffult to read and learn.

Then the doctor came round and I said "I seem to be helf witted". "Oh no" she said "You just had a small stroke. We can help you work hard." that was really good news. "Still", I though, "that was a small stroke what a big one can be like?" I learned that when I was able to talk a little with the other patents.

As to working hard - I only start. I had been always a fast learner if I was really had some interresting to do, and what could be more interresting than learning to talk and hear - to say and write and read. But was trying before I could run before could I could walk. By giving every moment for study I though, so to say, learn to speak Chinese in six weeks. But it doesn't work like that. The first lesson had to learn was patience - and the most difficult. Here I really have to thank all the people who helped me with my Speech Therapy. Patiencely but firmly they took me through the simple things that I needed to know first - Such as reading the clock and writing chjeques, when I wanted to take a part in the conversation and to read all the new books that had been published while I couldn't see them. The simple and relative boring I could pick up at any time. But my Speech Therpist insisted on doing first things first. It seemed sort of "Alice through the Looking Glass" system for me but it worked. While I was struggling with cheques I found I was talking - even if I was complaining about not faster.

After that things got slowly but steadly on. My good friend Betty and had a short holiday in Yujoslavia. The place and the weather were lovely but I was finding conversation diffcult, espially if when many people were talking at the same time. But last October we had a chance to get a trip to China. Of course I was a lot better than our last trip, but this was so fascinating that I couldn't think about how I had to speak - it just came out.

We had one English guide for the whole the trip and a new Chinese guide each time we stopped to see a new place. These were joung and pleasent - normally students. They urged us to ask as many questions as we wanted to, and I found that I could as many as the rest - and understand the answers too! I could even say how much I enjoyed talking to them and showing the places we had heard about. Whether it was because of that or not (once I have over the effect of Jet Lag), I could still talk a little better, and also I found that reading was going much easily. In fact I was reading for pleasure, just for practice. So that I got rather slow about writen this, because I had so many things I wanted to read.

THE EXPERIENCE OF APHASIA

> I have had to amit that reading will never good as it was but it will manage somehow to keep in contact and that is the important thing.

Mrs. H. 80 years old. Retired teacher of English as a foreign language. February 1987 (nearly two years after a stroke)

In 1977, when I was 29 years old, I had a cerebral haemorrhage. At the time, I was head of Write-Up in a factory, which is part of an international electrical group. I enjoyed going out with my wife, having a drink with my friends, and playing the organ in the local ballroom on Friday and Saturday nights.

I am now physically disabled. I am paralysed down the right-hand side of my body and I sometimes need to use a walking stick. In the beginning, (after the operation to stop the bleeding in my brain,) I couldn't speak at all, I couldn't understand what anybody said to me, and I couldn't recognise words, so I couldn't read or write. I only realised my wife was there by the feel of her wedding ring on her finger. Now, I still have quite a lot of bother with my speech - I can't always say what I want to say, and sometimes I can't follow what people say to me. It is much easier for me to understand what's going on on television because I've got the picture in front of me, to help me. With radio, it's hopeless, I can't follow it. It's funny, that! The telephone's much the same. it was very difficult at the beginning, and it still gives me some problems. I rely on seeing people when they're speaking - people give clues! That's how I can understand what's being said. I really need to see them face on, too. Because I have visual problems, if people sitting on my right side, speak to me, then I can't see them, and I can't make sense of what they are saying.

JUMBLY WORDS

I can speak well enought, make myself understood - I hope!! - and generally I can follow what people say to me. I can read, not complicated stuff like a novel, though I've tried, but I can manage newspaper headlines and short articles, and I can read what I've written, as long as I keep it simple. I can write quite well with my left hand and I can spell. I've learnt, with help, to do all these things again.

During the first few years after my operation I found out who my real friends were - these "real" friends were patient and understanding, and had the time to include me in what they were doing, and to bring me into their discussions and conversation.

Obviously, I'm more at ease with friends than with strangers; my friends don't confuse me or make me feel uncomfortable. They allow me time to get my words out, and they listen to what I have to say. I may pick up a couple of things in the wrong way, but usually they don't mind, and we have a laugh about it. They laugh with me, not at me. New people don't seem to know to treat me as a normal person; I think I'm normal, I feel normal, I am normal! Just because I can't speak like them and I look a bit different, they turn away, ignore me or speak to my wife or speak to somebody else.

I suppose, my problems are mostly in trying to make myself understood. People tend to finish off my sentences for me when I get stuck, and they usually end up with the wrong end of the stick. I get annoyed, and it can take a long time to sort things out again - if by then I've not forgotten what I was going to say in the first place! It's like getting tied up in knots!

There were times, particularly in the early stages, when I was in hospital that I wanted to give up. I was very depressed; I cried into myself when it was dark and no-one could see me. It was a mixture of not knowing what would happen, where I was going, what I was going to do, or if I would get better. I was crying inside; I couldn't let anyone see how I felt; I had to put

THE EXPERIENCE OF APHASIA

on a brave face; I was afraid - it was real fear - I felt I was neither here nor there, just flotsam and jetsam, that was it! I was just a nobody; decisions were taken for me, and my feelings didn't seem to come into it. It was difficult for me to express them anyway! "They" decided what they were going to do, regardless of what I thought. It is still so clear in my mind. I tried to speak to "them", but all that came out was jibberish! I knew what I wanted to say, what I wanted to tell them, but I couldn't get it out. It frightened me. I thought I'd be like that for ever and ever. I remember I was really chuffed when I was allowed home for the first time. I knew I could manage, but I don't think "they" were so sure. A decision was made at 2.30 pm. on Friday afternoons when the consultant and his troop came round; you'd be on tenderhooks wondering if you'd be allowed home. It was terrible. I know they were only doing their best for me, but they seemed to ignore me, as I was the last to be told. I didn't like going home for the weekend and having to come back to hospital on Sunday night. It was great to be going home; home was normal; hospital was false somehow. It felt like coming back to prison!

Even when I was improving I often felt like chucking it in. People kept on at me ..... on and on and on! Some people more than others! I often felt "what's the point". but I realise now that if they hadn't gone on at me, I wouldn't be where I am to-day, and I certainly wouldn't have been able to do any of this.

My wife has had to bear the brunt of having a disabled husband, but what I don't need is sympathy; I can do things round the house - I do them every day. I'm the house-wife now!! We've got a dog, (we got her about 6 months after my operation) and she makes me go out in all kinds of weather. She's a lovely dog, and she's a real companion to me. We go abroad every year on holiday; I love the sun and flying! I've even been on a camping holiday in France. I go shopping on own, coping with the buses, swing doors and shop assistants!! The first time I went shopping on my own (about 16 months after my illness) was to get something for my wife's birthday. I didn't tell her. I wanted it to be a surprise. My Speech Therapist knew as we'd talked about it and planned it together. I had to catch a bus into the town, cross a busy road, walk along a side street into a shop to use their escalator to get down to another street level, and then I was O.K. My wife phoned me up from her work - she phoned three times, and when she got no reply, she got really anxious. She phoned the next door neighbour who went into the house, and reported back that there was no-body there but the dog. The fourth time she phoned, she got me. I was given a "rocket", and how! It spoiled my surprise just a bit! But I'd done it, and I felt great. Looking back, I think I was pretty courageous too! I don't like asking people for help unless it's really necessary. I like to be independent.

I think perhaps, that young people have the most trouble accepting me. They seem embarassed by my disabilities and cover this up by ignoring me completely. Other people of my own age and older are usually helpful, but it just depends. It's the blank looks, being treated as if I were stupid, as if I'm not quite right in the head, and even the odd hostile glance, that gets me. I'm very aware of how people react to me, and it's not just them, it's me too. I get a funny feeling at the nape of my neck; I can feel these eyes boring into my back as I walk out of a shop or into a resturant. I always know when someone is looking at me.

I know that in a way, I limit the behaviour of people around me and I don't mind up to a point, being ignored or left out, but as long as I feel that I can have my say occasionally and am included, then I'm fairly happy and content with my life.

I've been very lucky all the way along ... I've had the help of my wife, the speech therapist, and the physiotherapist. I had physiotherapy for 2 years

THE EXPERIENCE OF APHASIA

- I know the exercises I'm supposed to do but I don't always do them! I still have speech therapy. I went to the Art therapist for a while and that was great because I've always liked drawing, and it was just him and me. He was the same age as me and we used to talk about football - we used to argue about it! And we'd talk about things that just men talk about.

I've had a lot of help putting all this down on paper. I couldn't have done it myself; it's taken ages to do! I've had most of the ideas, but I've needed someone to put them together for me. There's a lot more I could say, but I think I've done enough for the moment.

On the whole, I've learnt to come to terms with myself. Everyone deserves the chance to be accepted for themselves.

Jim

Chapter 4

ADAPTATION

"A way of life changed in a minute of time."

My husband had a severe stroke at the age of 66 in May '83. He was left quite disabled and returned home after 10 weeks in hospital.

It is not the care he needs for his physical disability that is the hardest part - I could cope with that fairly well - it is the absolute loss of speech. As he also gets gestures wrong it is all rather distressing for both of us. We are lucky that he can read a certain amount, but cannot put letters together to write words.

Of course I know his everyday needs, but he was a man who loved talking to people and he still wants to tell me what happened at the Day Centre or the people he has seen, and mostly I haven't a clue. If I know his train of thought sometimes I strike lucky, but anything coming out of the blue is hopeless.

He had Speech Therapy for some months but although he enjoyed it all, it was discontinued through lack of progress.

Until one has first hand experience of such a handicap it is impossible to realise the trauma involved.

I wondered if the enclosed poem might be of some interest to you - we can only guess at the patient's feelings, but this might sum it up in a small way.

JUMBLY WORDS

We took it for granted day by day
That hours would pass in the usual way -
Small talk and arguements - a way of life
So well known to a husband and wife.
Taken for granted the gift of speech,
With never a thought of the loss of each -
Communication and telling of news,
No more discussions or exchange of views.
A way of life changed in a minute of time
Just gestures and sounds with no sense of rhyme.
Locked in a world of thoughts and ideas
With no way of sharing, but laughter and tears.
Just left with a future with hope as the key
That one of these days
They will **understand** me!

Christine Bayliss

THE EXPERIENCE OF APHASIA

He sits in that same spot
How many hours? How many remaining days?
What does he see? What does he think?
What occupies a mind for so many hours?
He seems so numb, so helpless.

It is only me that interrupts this calm
and introduces conflict.
Conflict, when facts are forced into the open.
When reality is faced head on and no allowance made.
"Profound impairment in all modalities".

And yet, there's a calmness, an understanding
founded on trust and true fellow feeling.
How I feel for that man - I feel I know him,
That he knows I understand.

How much can I do? How much do I know?
When he smiles all is peaceful and hope survives.
But when that calm turns to raging, stormy madness
What can be done to help?
Nothing can be done for one who is so anguished?

And yet the times of trust and confidence encourage.
Insistent hope cautiously urges me on.
What can I do to help this man regain all that he has lost?
- his window on the world so cloudy.
Can it ever become clear?

Perhaps the scene will fall into focus.
Perhaps the awful confusion will lift
(and life can be lived) with experiences to be added
Instead of a distorted revision of the past.

I feel responsible.
In one man's world, perhaps the only beam of light.

What is he thinking now, as I sit here wrapped in my own thoughts
and incriminating his?
I can see him sitting head in hand.
The posture of a despairing old man.
But he's not! He's young and oh so painfully alive.

And what of his innocent and trusting wife?
She looks on with the eyes of a mother .....
and blushes with pride at his success
and scolds with curt annoyance his failures
- that are just too inevitable.

When, "do you want the bottle?" becomes the only interaction
All dignity and responsibility is gone.
The man is left bereft
(of all the things that made him)
The man he still is inside.

THE EXPERIENCE OF APHASIA

> We will persevere.
> Life will become more meaningful.
> And perhaps more painful.
> But at least he's feeling .... and feelings must find expression.

Written by a newly qualified Speech Therapist.

"A very frequent and most unreserved correspondence"

The correspondence which I am about to describe was carried out over many years with a particular group of dysphasic men. They had a number of things in common. All had suffered strokes leading to severe dysphasia during their fifties when they were at the height of their careers. All were very well educated and well read and each of them was engaged in work which centered upon communication. Not only were their working ives dominated by the necessity to express and to communicate but they were all sociable men who delighted in conversation, repartee and the companionable exchange of ideas. In each case, the effect of dysphasia was the profound disruption, not only of a prosperous career but of a whole way of life.

I met each of these men for the first time as his speech therapist. They represented one section only of my clinical population, the sophisticated language user who is above all interested in regaining control of language and through it expressing the person he was and still feels himself to be. My clinical contacts lasted for periods of around two years during the intensive phase of rehabilitation and were prolonged for months or years during the phase of maintenance and readjustment. My correspondence has been of much longer duration and in the case of two of them can be measured in decades.

Our correspondence first started during holiday periods when postcards would arrive at the clinic, first written by the spouse and signed by the patient and then written by the patient himself. "Having a glorious time. Talking quite well"; and on a later occasion, "Very beautiful weather. Be back on the 13th". Another patient was less fortunate. "We went to Tintagel and inspected the rain". Our rehabilitation work together involved both the spoken and the written word since both were equally affected. In the case of the visitor to Tintagel, the importance of writing became paramount when he and his wife decided to emigrate to Australia. Any contact with English friends would have to depend upon letters. Consequently I received my first epistle, a couple of months before departure.

"Forgive me but I must practice on you ... and without a dictionary." However, honesty compels the addition of an asterisk in the following line together with a footnote "dictionary". Three months later he achieves a letter of one and a half pages written on board ship and without a dictionary. It is not an easy task. "P.S. I takes me an hour (approx) to write its. Gin and tonic are 1/- ... that helped me!"

The next year shows great progress. "In the meantime I've got a job in the income tax office and I can add up quite nicely. I have been at it for 4 months now and I can keep up with the "blokes". I'm quicker at reading ... books and newspapers ... and I still can't spell. Writing you is a labour of love."

This labour of love continued until the writer's death with the letters becoming increasingly informative. Although they were not the fluent and

THE EXPERIENCE OF APHASIA

lengthy or crisp and cogent communications that he would have been able to write before his stroke, they were well able to convey the nature of his own life in Australia and to enquire after mine. Our correspondence was no longer concerned entirely with the here and now, as is evident from his response to learning that I was proposing to go to the Passion Play at Oberammagau. "I should think its Commercialised appallingly ... films whizzing and blaring ... when I was there it was more sedate. Occasionally the yanks would click their camera's but that is all."

Another writer showed very early in our correspondence, the ability to surmount any preoccupation with his own handicap and use the letter to maintain the social conventions. His letter to me upon the death of my mother could hardly be improved upon for warmth and directness. "... terribly grieved that you have lost your mother. What will you do with your father? Our sympathy to you all."

This writer became very skilled at picking up my wording to continue the theme. "David and you have been to see your father. I am glad David have been a wonderful companion." He also uses a telegraphic style most vividly to tell of his own experiences. "Went to hear the Haydn concerto played by Rostropovich and Britten conducting. Out of this world!!! Marvellous!! Very thrilling." The content here belies the effect of naivete which is the almost inevitable result of language loss. The writer, or speaker, cannot handle language in a complex enough manner to convey nuance and fine shades of meaning. Each of my dysphasic correspondents tends to rely heavily upon the exclamation mark in default of the ability to employ an elaborate sentence or make use of a qualifying phrase. However, the message is certainly conveyed and communication is maintained. Indeed, to a recipient already touched by the courage, tenacity and effort that have gone into the letter, the errors are more endearing than technically flawless constructions would be. "Thank you exceedingly much for the nice card and the message."

In one instance, the correspondence was initiated by the patient in the attempt to come to terms with his state. Dated December 2nd, it proceeds "this year you have been very kind in helping me to recover so well from my stroke in January. Now it seems to be stabilized or improvements are very small indeed! I know that there are some functions that I will never recover properly again. Never-the-less I hope that I will see you in 1979, for a check-up say ever three months so I can try hard to improvement by your criticism and your encouragements."

Writing at the beginning of Febnruary to make his appointment he puts ".... so I suggest that Tuesday, 20th February at 9 a.m. as a firm appointment, and I hope that will be convenient also! That he now if it isn't please."

This last sentence makes interesting reading and betrays the writer's remaining difficulty in converting a sound pattern to a written one. He must surely have intended to write "Let me know if it isn't, please." While a speech therapist can make the appropriate deduction, such errors will cause confusion in ordinary social correspondence, particularly when they appear amid an otherwise fluent and accurate paragraph. The writer continues to make the point that he sees his present difficulties as minimal. "I am so well now, in physical and also in spiritual that my life today is good in however way, and the small inability is nothing at all."

(Another letter that month accompanies a present.)

"I told you on Tuesday this week about the book I was tried to buy, but the reprint was delayed. Yesterday the order gave in and I therefore sent it to you right away." The book in question was an anthology compiled by Robert Morley of "Bricks" of the conversational variety; those infelicitous

THE EXPERIENCE OF APHASIA

remarks which sometimes arise when attention is not fully upon the subject or the listener. The book was sold to benefit autistic children and was chosen by my friend to remind me of him. "The children have a benefit too and that is nice."

Many of my intelligent dysphasic correspondents were able to indicate that they were well aware of how they must appear to others. The "Book of Bricks" shows that the giver well appreciated that he was insufficiently in command of his own tongue. A similar insight though of a slightly different nature was shown by another dysphasic man whose difficulties also lay in the area of verbal analysis, albeit rather more severely. Although his comprehension was severely impaired he retained, to an extraordinary extent, his interest in words. The following extract is taken from a journal paper but I hope I may be allowed to use it again since it is a particular favourite of mine.

Topic: The latest exploration of Space

Use has been made of language formulas governed by the expressions, "How long?", "When?", "What?" and others. Vocabulary had been extended by use of words "galaxy", "constellation", which had directed attention to synonyms. Upon Mr. K's recalling the rhyme "Twinkle, twinkle little star". the therapist responded with the more erudite version:

> "Scintillate, scintillate, globule vivific,
> Fain would I fathom thy substance specific
> High up above in the ether capacious,
> Strongly resembling a gem carbonaceous."

55

JUMBLY WORDS

This appeared to be new to Mr. K. who asked for it to be repeated and then written down. After a moment's study he observed, "Oh, they are the same, they are the same thing!" Then, not quite accurately but perfectly intelligible, "Oh well, a nod is as good as a wink to a blind horse."

The last communication I had from Mr. K. was a particularly nice one. "Here on a visit to see our first grandson."

Looking over these letters, and the many others which I have collected and connot bring myself to throw away, I am aware of the way my own feelings have changed. In the immediacy of the correspondence I simply thought of the person. I pictured his situation, filled in the gaps, read between the lines and replied to the letters. Reading them across the years, I am struck by the very strong impression of personality which emerges from the imperfect writing. All the authors are struggling to maintain a way of life which had been bound up with language in all its manifestations. Instead of withdrawing from social intercourse and refusing to take responsibility for its maintenance, they work to keep these precious lines of communication open. In doing so, they both risk and learn to handle, confusion, misunderstanding and loss of dignity. It is worth underlining the fact that these letters were written during days when each man must have experienced equal frustration and fatigue through trying to communicate through the spoken word. In every case, difficulties with spoken language were just as severe as with written. The alternative of communicating by means of the telephone was no easier and, as we frequently corresponded across continents, it would have been impractically expensive for both parties.

There can be few more eloquent tributes to the power of the English language than these attempts by those who once commanded it, to use it again in this reduced but now, I think, impoverished form.

In addition to the correspondence maintained with dysphasic patients, I have saved many letters written by relatives and friends of the sufferer. Some of these, sadly, were replies to my own letters of condolence upon the death of their spouse or parent. They were not only kept to remind me of the patient but of what is important in therapy. This is not always clear at the time, particularly to the young clinician. If you see someone who is at first overwhelmed by a profound loss of all the routes through which communication is conveyed, you are continually aware of the inadequacy of what you, as a speech therapist can offer. This was very much the case with a young woman of 32 who became aphasic following an embolism. During the months in which we worked together she was able to regain very little speech or writing and when I heard of her death from a second embolism, I was distressed to think of how sad her last months must have been for her and how little I had been able to do to help. The letter from the husband shows that he shares my views about effect on his wife's life.

"I can only say that I thought a great deal of _____ and would have accepted her no matter what. I think she would have preferred this way out."

The passage which follows showed me very clearly that therapy cannot only be measured in terms of function regained. Indeed, perhaps relatives who see the patient every day and can continually contrast his behaviour with what it once was, do not expect that the therapist will be able to restore this behaviour. Perhaps they are more concerned that the patient's spirit should be supported as much as possible.

"I most wish to tell you how much I have appreciated your kindness and help shown to _____ . Your unfailing help always gave _____ courage to carry on when things seemed hopeless to her."

Another letter shows a different kind of expectation, both from the patient and his family.

"....and thank you also for the great effort you made to help my father regain his speech. As you could see, he was a man who appreciated efficiency and he knew that he was making, with your guidance, the sort of progress which gave him hope."

The words that recur most frequently in the letters are "guidance". "help" and "encouragement".

"We are all comforted in the knowledge that he received so much encouragement from you during his long illness."

These letters have certainly played a considerable part in shaping the development of a clinician. They are continual reminders that the dysphasic person and his/her family live with the problem all the time. They are the ones who can measure what is going on in the way of communication and of changes in attitude.

"The communication side of living was his whole life until his illness and he was very quietly getting quite inconsolable about it till you started leading him along the way back."

The final extract is much longer than the others but it is particularly perceptive. it is taken from a letter written by a physician in response to one of mine. This physician had referred her own aunt to me for private speech therapy following a cerebral catastrophe leading to a profound aphasia affecting all modalities. My letter was written in the attempt to get more help for the aunt but also contained an apologia for the little that I had been able to achieve. The reply is extremely helpful:

"My own feeling is that she really is making a tiny bit of progress in that she sometimes spontaneously brings out a necessary word and can read with some comprehension.

I feel that there can be do doubt that your treatment is an enormous help to her and she has repeatedly told me so herself. In fact, when we come back from .... she agitates to see you, actually repeating ... (which is an affectionate Russian version of your name) until told exactly when you are coming.

I do hope that you will not feel it too much of a burden to go on treating her, as I really believe that the vital part of the little progress she is able to make springs from the combination of faith in herself and technique, that you are giving her.

She is getting much braver. This Saturday she managed to convey to me that she wanted to ask an old friend of mine to tea to meet her ... she is usually so reluctant to meet anybody outside of a few old friends who come again and again. I took the opportunity of getting several other people together and she thoroughly enjoyed it, managed to join in the conversation a bit and even brought out the words "paint" and "ago" in a desperate attempt to tell us the story of a portrait that an artist friend (who was there) had painted about 20 years ago."

The letter then deals firmly with what must have been a very frank and contrite remark of my own.

"I can't think why uou say that from the point of view of rehabilitation you are wasting my father's money. The central core of rehabilitation is precisely what you are doing: building up the patient's courage, interest and self confidence so that he can co-operate fully in regaining skills and adapting his damaged self to new ways of coping.

What you are doing for her in this way is most precious to us all so do continue if you possibly can."

The range of conditions encouraged under the term "dysphasia" and its degrees of severity is something for which the therapist can never be prepared during training. With the information and insight that accrues around each new case, you learn a little bit more about what to do and how to do it. The contribution of the patient's family is not only vital to the patient's progress and survival, but is extraordinarily helpful to the development and survival of the therapist.

Betty Byers Brown
Speech Therapist

These are two aspects of a remarkable woman - Sarah's grandmother and my mother. They are written both as a tribute to her, and to share the experience of trying to help a dysphasic person both personally and professionally.

Daughter

Two years ago my mother was a rather proud, obstinate, determined, occasionally procrastinating and humorous woman. She still is, despite a severe stroke leaving here severely dysphasic.

The week-end before this happened I had felt a heavy sense of unease: half a tooth fell out, and I twisted my ankle. I phoned her to say goodbye before a weeks' holiday in Majorca. "Lots of love" she said, and it was to be many weeks before I heard her speak again.

Forty-eight hours later I was involved in one of those nightmare sequences of events, trying to get back to England. A phone call had merely said my mother had been "rushed to hospital" after a severe stroke. My younger daughter collected me from Heathrow and we drove straight to see her.

I didn't know what to expect - I certainly didn't know what a stroke WAS - I had vague ideas of being struck down, paralysed, but the one thing I had never envisaged was that my articulate and clever-fingered mother would be doubly struck down, that she wouldn't be able to speak except in frightened gibberish, and that the whole of her right side would be paralysed. The memory of her eyes beseeching me to set the clock back, to get her out of the hospital, will never go away. At 88, she had never been in hospital in her life.

Two unexpected difficulties presented themselves: it was hard to get anyone in the hospital to explain WHAT had happened, in layperson's terms, and secondly, I was strongly affected by my mother being so ill. I, who had had to deal competently in the past with illness and emergencies, found it extremely hard to realise that she might die. I felt unprepared and at the same time angry with myself for my ignorance and lack of readiness: I had fallen into the trap of believing my mother indomitable. I suppose I had thought that she might suddenly keel over one day, and that would be that. So I had to face what happened next.

There seemed not much desire on the hospital professional's part to impart information even to my natural response of wanting to be USEFUL and not merely an emotional, anxious relative. I think that lack of information, at the outset, contributed to my becoming, for a while, obsessional, really believing I could will my mother's speech back, that if I cared deeply enough, I could heal her.

My elder daughter helped me out of this morass. As a speech therapist she gave me as much information as she could, talking to me calmly, posting leaflets from the Chest, Heart & Stroke Association, and firmly divesting me of all the fantasies and hopes I held on to that my mother would, one day, speak clearly and naturally again.

We discussed how impeded we were as daughter and grand-daughter: Sarah found it hard to be professional with her grandmother, pity and compassion perhaps getting in the way of professional calm. At this stage and subsequently, so much could be done to enlist the relatives' support in whichever ways are most supportive to the patient AND the professional. Instead I met reluctance and sometimes felt I was interfering in asking questions, wanting to know routines and why they referred specifically to my mother.

This not being told also affected my mother, since she COULDN'T ask questions! She was not given explanations and in the early weeks she was talked over, never to, never given reasons, which seemed to add unnecessarily to her anguish. Throughout, whenever I sat down and explained things as best I could, she calmed down. Initially I could only offer her vague reassurances, but not until Sarah gave me, steadily and repeatedly useful and relevant information, did I really understand what had happened, what could be improved and, more important, what could not, and then felt I could pass on this calmness to my mother - that, in fact, she could share in the truth about herself.

Some resentment and frustration still reside in her - and in me, as her daughter. For her, it is a question of why, why me, at the end of a long hard life, healthily lived. Why lose my speech and the use of my craftswoman's hands? For myself, I had always tried to get closer to my mother, and in some ways I feel she is even stronger in her dysphasia, and it's even harder to feel what she wants, and who she is.

But she battles on: when she first got out of hospital, she wept, and kept saying over and over, "want die, want die".

The other day, close to 90. she announced, clear as a bell, "Going to live to a hundred."

THE EXPERIENCE OF APHASIA

Grand-daughter's story

My father phoned late one night ... "Granny has had a stroke" ... the words took on a peculiar intensity over the phone. I was working as a Speech Therapist in the north of the country. My grandmother was living in the south. She was eighty eight at the time. Worse, my mother, who had been visiting her regularly for the last two years, had finally taken a short holiday. She was abroad, and I sensed her desperation, could see her trying to get back, her terrible feeling of guilt above all, because she was also abroad when her father died.

I remember looking around the hospital for a card to send to Granny. Nothing suited, and what do you send someone who's just suffered a big stroke and is dysphasic? In the end I sent her a hopelessly inappropriate one of two football players scoring a goal.

A few days later I met Granny. She looked lost, confused and very very vulnerable. I remembered the last time I'd seen her. We went for a drive and stopped at a farm shop, where Granny discussed all the different strains of local potatoes. We'd had tea and discussed the state of the world. She'd written and thanked me for the eighty eighth birthday present in her spidery handwriting. And here she was, obviously very dysphasic. I had always seen her in her own well known surroundings, so it was quite a shock.

It never worked, once I took on my professional role. Granny knew straight away and would instantly look put out. I remember on that first visit I patted her hand in a concilliatory automatic way and she whipped it away. Even then she was indicating her independence, pride and strength. I had never seen my mother so distraught, rushing round, hovering, ordering extra equipment, wanting the best, the most, for Granny. I remember telling her to take it easier - she had been getting up at the crack of dawn every other day, driving through London to Granny's home town, stopping off for coffee at my place on the way home and looking so tired. Yet somehow it was imperative to herself that she stay "together" in front of me.

My mother is very interested in people, communication, writing, talking and hence the condition of dysphasia. I explained, alongside the Speech Therapist seeing Granny. And explained more, counselled her and the rest of the family, and realised in the process how, when talking to a very receptive (but anxious) person, you need to say things again, and several times, before someone is able to absorb the impact and realisation occurs. And Granny was changing. She was looking less bewildered, recovering some of her "self", her comprehension was improving and she was no longer relying on her own and others facial expressions to give and receive meaning. She was also becoming more demanding because she was more in control.

She moved home, with nursing care ... a few phrases were emerging, some very poignant ... "She thinks I'm deaf" (her cleaning lady); "It's so prustrating". The rest was sentences begun but not finished, some rather bizarre sentences, e.g. "There's a lot of lovely truffles" when trying to talk about tatting. She had previously done some very beautiful knitting, crochet and tatting, including a crocheted bedspread. Her hands would wave in circles in the air or were thumped on arms of chairs. But she kept trying, keeps trying to this day. She has tremendous will-power and strength of spirit. I felt some of her frustration and despair. I was also discovering new aspects of her character I'd never known about. When I'd seen her before her stroke it was very much in the role of visiting grand-daughter (which I still am!), seeing her social, well groomed exterior. In fact, as I got to know her better, ironically, after her stroke, I realised I hadn't know her all that well previously.

THE EXPERIENCE OF APHASIA

I found keeping to my role of grand-daughter worked the best for Granny and I. But I continued to experience guilt because I wasn't "doing more" professionally.

My mother was taking on most of the responsibility for Granny's welfare. She needed to let go a bit, to go on a holiday - there was still this tremendous feeling of self control from her. My sister and I booked two holidays, but something always seemed to crop up with Mum, to prevent them. Then a friend whisked her off on a weeks' holiday. She came back, her whole face different.

Then Granny moved to a residential home. I remember that day, the visual tableaux of Granny, my mother and I, etched permanently in my mind: we had packed Granny's things in the car. She appeared remote and almost unconcerned, yet was leaving a place she had lived in for thirty years or more. At the last minute she wanted to take her pot of African violets, so I picked it up and we left. Granny never looked back.

"The Other Viewpoint"

As the wife of one disabled by a stroke I would like to put forward some views for the appraisal and possible consolation for those in a similar position.

Of all the afflictions effected by a stroke I feel the loss of speech to be the most frustrating and debilitating for both patients and their spouses. Try as one may to exercise the patience and understanding expected of one there are times when I personally have felt I could take no more and I consider lack of the former not one of my shortcomings.

The understanding is perhaps just as difficult because as we all know one has to experience in order to fully understand. In doing ones best therefore, a little self pity creeps in on realising the patient is equally unable to comprehend your position. The old vicious circle!

At the beginning my husband would not speak at all, then when able to cope with "yes" or "no" he said one when he meant the other. He reversed the gender and still often does. So "he" became "she" and vice versa. One would have to show the object of which one was speaking, for example. Even now after three and a half years one often has to write a word, here and there, on paper for it to be understood.

Now of course with the admirable aid and compassion of the speech therapists as well as Mother Nature, my husband can converse with me and I don't feel so alone any more. Humour too has helped ease the situation. This has come about because my husband has found the will to make himself do things, like clock repairing, typing - also wine making and now of course, he is editing a newsletter, "Orange Box". This has given him the confidence required to go on from strength to strength.

I have hitherto dealt only with speech but because of Arthur's many other physical disabilities we are not able to go out often. I often suggest that we should go out and drive through the Devon scenery which he loves so much, but I get a negative reply. Our son has taken us for the occasional drive which we enjoy all the more because it is an event for us.

One has to understand the reason for this hermit-like attitude in my husband - the reason for his reluctance is that he fears should the car break down I would not be able to cope and he can do nothing now. This I understand and so cannot push too hard. If one is going on to the moors or wherever we go, inevitably one either wants to walk and explore and the patient knows this is not possible, then to avoid the temptation and resultant frustration, the sensible course is to refuse to go .....

I have touched lightly and sparingly on most of the problems because inevitably individuals differ and some will have problems that others do not.

THE EXPERIENCE OF APHASIA

Also I mustn't give my husband too much to type.
Good luck and best wishes to all who share similar problems.

Vera West. Written 4 years after her husband's stroke.

I am a disabled person now in my 70th year. In May 1985 I had a stroke, which left me entirely speechless, a traumatic experience in any age group.

Originally, in my religion I was a public speaker and reader and to be suddenly rendered speechless was horrifying.

Amid the copious tears I managed to reach my phone for a friend as I was alone at the time. At these times I realized the value of prayer, and I was determined to read again as soon as was possible.

I joined my local stroke group and asked for homework, now, in December 1986 I am able to read again in an hour long discussion, memory is not too good and the mind goes blank, spelling is not too hot yet. I took the advice of the speech therapist and took up drawing and water colour painting to rid myself of the frustration of trying to find words to express myself. I owe everything to the group therapists.

Ron Hudson

(One of Ron's pencil sketch's is reproduced on the next page.)

JUMBLY WORDS

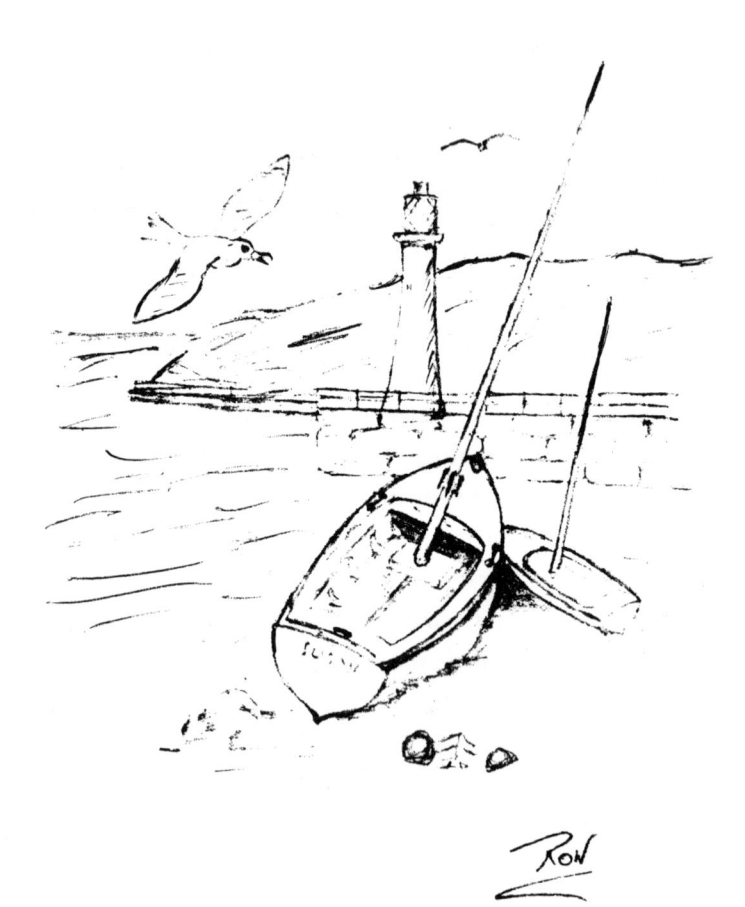

THE EXPERIENCE OF APHASIA

Living with Dysphasia

The cause of my problem was said to be an embolism which entered my brain at the time of a by-pass operation to replace three faulty arteries and mend one. X-ray scans failed to find an embolism or any hole in my brain where it might have been. Whatever the cause, dysphasia was real enough. When I was in the Intensive Care ward, it was said that I was very agitated and I had to be given a jab to calm me down.

In the ordinary ward it seemed to me that I was the same as other patients. We all slept restlessly at night; we got out of bed and sat in a chair, then back in bed and so on. In the day I was soon walking up and down the corridors which other patients did not seem to do. When I got home I was restless at night in the same way and every time I woke up I had a nightmare. This situation lasted about five months.

From the time I left hospital until Christmas, a matter of about four months, I had no idea of what was happening at home nor do I remember anything. There was one exception; this was a day out to another town for a wedding.

A shock came to me when I went to the local school where my grandchildren go, for a carol concert and I realized for the first time that I had a problem. Music had no meaning to me; no way could I sing. During the intervals teachers made jokes which I did not understand; the audience laughed their heads off and I didn't know why! I felt isolated and depressed. I felt the same at Christmas when presents were being opened and games were being played without me.

I usually like to take slides at family events, but I found I could not load my camera. My son bought me another one which I did manage to load, reasonably easily; later on when I had got much better, I tried the first camera again. What a surprise I got when I found no problem in loading it whatever.

During this period and later, much annoyance and exasperation took place between my wife and me. Accordingly arrangements were made for me to attend speech therapy. I cannot recall attending the first sessions nor can I remember the therapist writing some advice for both of us, but as it was pinned up on the kitchen wall I know it had been written; it proved very useful.

During the day I had no need to bother about time; at night in bed I did like to know what it was. When my wife came into bedroom to say good night I would ask what time it was, she would tell me but I would disagree; she said the problem could be that it was a twentyfour hour clock. It did not seem to be this because when I got up in the night to go to the toilet I looked at the clock and noted the time. After a few minutes I came back and found the time was two hours later. I thought no way could I have spent all that time in the toilet!

I tried to work out percentages on a pocket calculater without success. I tried drawing; I could manage a square but some months later I still could not draw a cube. 1 I was able to play card games like patience, crib and canasta, provided I didn't try to score! On the other hand, I was unable to read. My main occupation was playing patience. When the weather allowed I would cycle around the local parks and perhaps go as far as Brentford and look at the Thames.

When I went shopping to a corner shop I had to point to what I wanted and describe the amount with my hands and I paid by displaying my open purse. In this situation and when I was asked questions in the street, I was very glad to have the card issued by the Chest, Heart & Stroke Association.

In order that I should be able to enjoy television programmes my wife and son bought a new television set which had subtitle facilities. This helpled, but not much at first because even this did not allow me to fully enjoy programmes. The old television is now fixed up with the word processor which I use to write this report.

It took some time before I could understand talk, for instance when my wife asked me questions she had to write them. I looked at them and spent a long time writing the response. My spelling was not too good either.

I had to attend the hospital quite a lot, two or three times a week; each time my wife came with me and spoke for me and proceedings were always very pleasant, except for waiting in the out-patients!

When I went for a ride in a car the passengers would chat happily while I sat there not understanding a word. This went on for some time because although I could understand people talking to me only, cross talk I could not. (I felt wonderful when one day I discovered that I could understand what people around me were saying, whatever the subject.)

The cross talk problem affected how people thought about me. I have been a member of a scientific society for some years. When I attended the January meeting, six months after the operation, I could not understand a word. I left before the end of the meeting. The same happened for the February meeting. After this I decided not to attend until the new session. The consequence of this was that the members thought I was deaf and decided to cross me off the committee. Imagine their surprise when I went back and I could now understand what they were saying. The result was I got my old job back.

By March I began to understand what people were saying, but it was patchy. For instance, I attended an all-day meeting on industrial chemistry. In the morning session I understood not a word, chemistry nor chit-chat in the coffee break. The afternoon session was quite different. It started with a talk about the Society and I understood it. The technical session dealt with physical chemistry with which I am familiar, as it is the subject I taught at the University. I understood everything. I felt delighted as I thought I had suddenly got better. But no, I understood no talk as people left the meeting nor when I got home. It was very depressing.

When I went to the University to see my friends I had a similar experience. I seemed to comprehend a long joke whereas the other listener did not. I also a friend of another lecturer was talking about the use of a Spectrum computer to send Morse code messages all over the world. I talked to him about the technical details and seemed to ask appropriate questions. One topic discussed why messages sent to New Zealand ended up in Brazil!

In the middle of March I went to a concert and I could hear and comprehend the music. I cried.

Another problem was writing. When I tried to write with a pen or pencil I made a mess. I had to use the word processor although this was not easy. What I wrote could also be nonsense although I was blissfully unaware of it. I sometimes still do.

I am a referee for the Royal Society of Chemistry and during March I received a chemical paper to look at and decide whether it should be published or not. I decided it should be and sent a report to the Editor. I often wonder what he made of it.

Now I am back in circulation. I am no more bothered by noise, at least no more than other people are, I can have a discussion although somtimes there is a hold-up while I search for a word. This is much better than it used to be. There was a time a few months ago when I got the names of my family mixed up, I knew that I was getting them wrong and this gave me a funny feeling.

Is it because I lost the sound of music that I now sing in a choir?

Robert Greenwood.

Chapter 5

RECOVERY

"I don't actually believe in the Resurrection ....
but there is something going on up there!"

On Wednesday 16th July it was a very hot sticky sort of day. I did my usual job of work. After tea I went to a committee meeting, arriving home approx 9.30pm. After a talk with my wife and son about what had been going on, I had my supper and we all went to bed. About 1/2 past 1-2 o clock I came down stairs unable to sleep being very hot. I went to the toilet came indoors and sat on the settee. I remember my wife coming down stairs to see where I had got to, although I knew all that she said to me, I could not communicate with her. She phoned the Dr and got an ambulance, the doctor said that I was to go to hospital. I still understood what they were saying and which hospital they were taking me to. The ambulance man was talking and reassuring me every thing was all right and telling me which roads and route we were taking. I remember also arriving at the hospital going on a trolley and a lady doctor trying to ask me questions, which I still could not answer, words would not come.

I did not know what was wrong with me, I thought about heart trouble as I had slight heart trouble since I was born, then I cannot remember anything more until I woke up on the ward next to sisters desk. Whether they gave me anything to sleep or I passed out I do not know. I just remember people about, then my wife came and said about some suction marks on my chest, but I did not know how they got there or could not speak only nod my head yes and no. The second night I tried to get out of bed to go to the toilet my mind told me too but my body told me I could

JUMBLY WORDS

not and I landed in a pile on the floor. I thought there was people a lot worse than me and needed the nurses attention. I went for a lot of tests and Xrays, but what they were all for I do not know as no body had told me. It took me 3 weeks to understand that I had had a stroke, my wife said that I had a stroke but I still thought it was something else as they had only said some medical long words, and it was not until I had asked a young nurse who new me what the matter was and she sat down and explained to me that it ment a stroke. C.V.A.

The doctors never seem to have time to listen to you as by the time my mind had sorted out the words they had gone on to the next patient. Then they told me some other tecnical word, they said it was like going into a washing machine it confused and frightened me, luckly my sister in law was visiting at the time, and came down to the room with me and the nurses, it looked a very large frightening machine and as I do not like going into confined spaces, I did not know what to expect. The man who was there knew that I was a aux. coastguard and we had raised money for this CAT Scanner talked to me and told me all about what they were going to do which helped to put me a bit more at ease. I was lucky that the nurses knew of me called me names, I thought she was rude but after speaking to my wife, they found out if I got worked up into a temper they got more response from me. it was the same with friends when they visited me. They used to ask me things like (what did you have for dinner) if I could not say right away, they tried to change onto another subject, but I would not be satisfied until I had told them the answer to the first question. The annoying thing was I new what I wanted to say but the right words would not come. I used to say for instance PIG instead of PORK. the one word which used to come out every time for all sorts of things was PYJAMAS. why we just dont know.

The O.T. nurse and the sister on my ward lived together must have

THE EXPERIENCE OF APHASIA

disscused things and they made me ask for every thing, they found I had a way of getting to the answer. I started to pick up and got friendly with the men on my ward then they moved me into another ward with an old gentleman who slept nearly all the time and a Polish man, I started to go backwards again then, it upset me to be parted from people who were understanding me. The ward sister spoke to my wife about why I was not getting on, she told her it was because I was taken away from people who I was getting on well with, so they then moved me back with a couple of them who was still in, I then began to pick up again.

I had quite a number of falls as I was trying to tet on to quickly as I could only concentrate on one thing at a time. I was soon pulled to halt when I had to have a pump fitted for 24 hrs a day for 10 days, as I had a clot on my leg.

It was a long time before I could concentrate on watching T.V. programme or read a paper approx 4-5 weeks it took a while to read something, some times going over the same words several times before they made any sence. It was then Bank Hiliday weekend in Aug when they decided to move me to another hospital but I was only there a week as it depressed me so much, as they were all very elderly and dying all the time. They were also doing some work on the ward putting in new windows. The physotherapy was very good at this hospital but there was no speech therapy at all. I was now at home and they soon found out I was getting depressed at not having any speech therapy so then was when they tried to get me moved to a new hospital.

I made good progress there with my speech as I was mixing with people and getting very good attention with the speech therapist. I am still having falls as I still can only concentrate on one thing at a time. Its made a great help being in this hospital especially on days when my leg play up, as I have to go down for my meals and departments. Although there are several stroke patients we all have different problems especially with speech. I now have found if I cannot say a word I can usually find an alternative one and I have to think before I speak. When I am with the speech therapst I get uptight and find I can use the languemaster better in my room on my own. I find I have problems with numbers, lower cased letters and days and time.

I find the computer a great help as there are discs which I can use and do it in my own time and pace.

It is all very frustrating, as I know all I want to say or write but not being bale to do it. Another annoying thing is that I still cannot use my call sign which I have to use when using Amature Radio, which took me 18 months of night school to get the call sign, now it just will not come out.

Terry Scott

To live or die

Well it all started when i was about 3 or 4, when i noticed that i had a tremor in my right hand. I remember going in the doctors and my mum would ask, if there was anything wrong, and she was told that i was being a spoiled little kid. So my mum believed him.

When i was about 7 or 8 or maybe 9 or 10. My sister and i took violin lessons at school. The teacher asked me if i had anything wrong because my tremor was realy bad, and i said no.

About a year later when my sister had left that school, i think the music teacher saw my social worker.

Later we got a letter through the door from the social worker, and she putils in contact with St. Peters Hospital

THE EXPERIENCE OF APHASIA

I had an appointment at the hospital and my social worker took me. When we amved there we had to go up the escalator then we asked somebody where the doctor was. Then we walked along the comdor and told the lady my name and sat down. Then a nurse came along and called my name and i took a deep breath, and followed the nurse into the room. The doctor said good afternoon and we just talked. He tested my reflexes, looked in my ears and asked if i could move everything. We sat down and started talking, and he said about having an operation where they would shave some hair off my head while i was still awake. Next he would drill a hole and after that they would put a tube-thing into my head. I said "no-ways" then he told me to change my hand towrite with my left hand. Then we went.

A couple if years later i noticed that my hand was getting worse and i could not wear high heeled shoes. Ialso noticed that in typing i had the embarasment of having to put my hands on topof the typewriter and i felt really akwaed because everyone was looking and my right was shaking. The teacher said "oh" away he walefs.

I was in my early teens, when i had to be seen at another hoseital. I didnt want to go into hospital because i knew there was sometwing wrony wieh me. So i has the tests done, Thae meant i hadto stay in hospil overhight. I had a bath put on a special guwn, and got into bed. Then the nurses came round and gave me an injection to help me sleep. 2 men came pushing a trolley and i was lifted on to the trolley. Iwas taken downstars by lift and they took me into this room and lifted me onto anotes table. Then he asked has my am when i woke up back in my bed on the ward. In the morning an ambulance came after breadfast and fook me back to the first hospital.

Mum decided i should have the operation.

The next day i woke up early and has a bath and washed my hair. I

JUMBLY WORDS

GOT IN BED, has the injection, and wait. Then they ware wheeling me over and taken down to the operating theatre, much later i was asleep.

I woke with a bandage round my head. Later i went back on the ward and i felt perfect my arm was beetter and my leg was better.

Some time later they took the stitches out of the left side of my head.

Then they said they would do the second operation. After that operation i found i could not move my fight arm and leg and my face felt frozen on that side. When looked to the left i could see but when i tried looking to my right i saw double.

II could hear what people were saying i could undertand them, but when i tried to speak it all came out ibbity jibbity. Stitches were taken out again in a different place. I as in a wheel chair.

After Christmas i was back in the ward far a night and then sent to the rehabitation centre next door to the hospital.

In the rehabilitation centre we did exercises. Physiotherapy and speech therapy. After some time i came to this school and i am still here at the age of 19 years. My dog is my best friend. I dont trust anyone because i have been let down a lot of times, my dog is the only triend ive got. I hope to be able to manage on my own and become a pop star.

Anon (19 year old girl)

THE EXPERIENCE OF APHASIA

At our stroke club last Friday one of the discusion was a book being written about stroke.

I would like to suggest that 4 years since the stroke I would like to go back to hospital to see the spicialist for a check up, as I feel much bitter in myself, an he could look me over, an I would understand, which would improve my status, although my Doctor is very good. I still think a second opinion would be useful.

R.D. Thair
December 1986

What is it like to have dysphasia?

There are four people. I was one of them. These other three people were talking to/at each other. They did not talk to me. They did not listen to me. They did not ask me anything. For two hours and a half.

   I **had this**! It was too much!
   And these were people that I knew for years.
   What is it like? DYSPHASIA ???

It was February 13th 1986 (Thursday)
I woke, and it was "funny".
I did not know this, of course, but I had a stroke.
I could see, so I got up and dressed, and went down stairs.
I know now that I was told that I had to go back up to bed.

JUMBLY WORDS

Suppose I went to the doctor and said that I have an **ache**. (a tooth-ache or ear-**ache**) The doctor says, I can't **see** it!
What is it like! **Show** it too me!

It is like the doctor. I can't listen, or read, or write or speak, but I can't show it or see it.

I was trying to think what is this word that am saying. I had a **long** try, and **then** I knew what the word is. But I couldn't say it.

I know! it's "IN-AD-IK-WET" - "INADIKWET". So I looked at the dictionary. I was right.

I felt **inadequate**, of everything, but in particularly, because by now I should have been able to know my meaning(s). At least, when I know a "WORD" I don't say "IT"

   I say - good gracious!
   or - What next!
   or - Oh dear!

I am thinking!
I had a stroke.
It was February. Now it is August.
I am getting better - but it takes a long time
Now it is December. I am getting more better (I hope). It is just about eleven months that I had the stroke, but I know that it will be longer yet.

I don't actually believe in the Resurrection, but I do think there is something going up there!

(December)

THE EXPERIENCE OF APHASIA

Problems

It is bad enough for people like me, who had a stroke, to learn to speak, and read and write again.

For instance, some people speak far too quickly for me, and also writing, too. (And also for some other people too).

Of course, there are some people who speak and write "scribble", but I am not talking of this.

It is not their fault if I don't know what I want to say, but they could speak slowly and clearly, what they are saying, and again, if they have to.

Notlikethis, orlikethat (too quickly)

Just   like   that. (slowly)

But   not   like   this   or   that.

How do people react?

Most of the people who I know are (were) (what is the word) sad? to say that I had (have) a stroke. Over this year, people say that I am getting better each month, but they know, like me, that it takes time.

They are good friends.

One man said "It is all in the mind!!" "It should be better now!!" (This was eight months ago.)

I wouldn't "wish" anyone to have a stroke. If "he" did, he would know very quickly that it was all in **His** mind.

(I hope that he never has one.)

JUMBLY WORDS

I (did) not know what I was saying or thinking! In fact, I couldn't say or think what, who, how, where or why of anything.

In particularly, WHY!? What did I **do**! Something I did, or said, I suppose! Ah well! I'll get **well** soon, and then I can **tell** every-one "What **was** It Like" when I had dysphasia.

If I had to ask - "What do you desire!?" I know!
It is un-dysphasia or dis-dysphasia. (It is a "new" word)

John Graney

Doctors and speech therapists have given me encouragement, and in the past, said that my speech was locked up in a chest and all we have to find is that key. It was so difficult to express the feelings and sensations I experienced as I went through dysphasia. For me, it is like a tree of wisdom which has been uprooted, dismembered bit by bit, branches, leaves and fruit, and that the trunk has been totally severed. Like a trunk, branches, leaves, roots and fruit, words and phrases float around in my head, as though they are all hidden behind opaque folds, some thicker and less accessible than others. I hope this has crystalized my feelings, since it was the predominant ambience in which I found myself. However, now that I have just described these feelings, I am able to smile more genuinely. Perhaps the sowing is taking place and growth potential is materializing.

In the first few days of dysphasia, I could not speak logically. My sister witnessed me telling my doctor that I was on my way to Spain with two sausages. I had been actually on my way to the dentist, taken two capsules for the headache. Funnily enough, I somehow managed to get the shape and number right. With the intensification of pressure on the left hemisphere, accompanied by expressionless eye contact, and a terrible feeling of being encapsulated in a black bottomless pit, I understood simple questions, but could not answer them. I introduced my brother as my sister and my mother as my uncle. Once I was tested by a speech therapist, the ugly reality came home to me. At that time, it was as though my net of words had been ostracized and banned to another unknown recess of my mind, and on recalling words I could only remember perhaps their stems. Naturally, my speech was very slow and I seemed to gesticulate more, especially when I was on my own, and set a cupped hand in front of my face as though I were waiting for a word to fall into it. In the middle of a conversation, I frequently searched the word I required, and if I dared to do so, then the word usually eluded me and the whole train of thought disappeared. If I attempted to ask people to repeat things twice or three times, I used to be none the wiser and return to that black pit. Progression with time and effort has been the hallmark of dysphasia, I think. I am now able to follow a general conversation a bit better. With no exaggeration, I am elated when an old familiar word floats unexpectedly into my mind, especially if it conjured up old events, like a flash-back, and that word and everything associated with it would slide into a more accessible area for future use. Apparently, my speech is more competent in conversation with others, but I still feel that my speech is not deep-seated in my mind and I cannot re-tell what I have just said, if I am successful, then it is with difficulty.

In reading, I could understand two lines at best and no more. Any more and my mind could not cope, I would be lost. With time, I began to undertstood and ingest bigger chunks of text and retain that information in my mind, but only fleetingly. In order to assimilate more information, even the gist of text, I somehow had to dupe my mind by reading quickly and uninterrupted - no fidgeting, not even turning the page over! From that point on, my reading improved. I still forget a lot of the material that I have just read and almost invariably, the main threads are scarcely retained. I must add that more successful reading depends on my interests, previous knowledge and understanding too. I always have a dictionary at my side to consult and to reassure myself that I have the correct meaning in mind. Sometimes words fit into a little rack as if it were to be used in a further game of scrabble. On other occasions, its futile. If I did not jot down the main points, then I would have great difficulty in remembering the main import. Having re-gained slightly improved reading capacity, I was inspired by the texts to think further. Unfortunately, (approx. 5/6 months later), abstract thoughts, ideas which were coming forward, were not so much a continuous flow of coherent, logical conclusions and questions, but rather a haphazard emergence of ideas etc. They were all circling somewhere in my mind, all vying to get out at once. If I become distracted in any way, even a glance in another direction, I could jeopardize the articulation of these ideas and feelings. Now 8 months on, I am beginning to get better at coming to a more decisive conclusion and have a slightly better management of thoughts.

Effort and striving towards an approachable and viable goal is a very positive incentive. Sometimes, I look upon my application to work (reading, listening to news etc.), as homework. It does have good results, even if it is on a long term basis. I do usually sense an improvement of one kind or another, and it brings a smile to my face and the realization that the previous inadequacies are becoming diluted. Sometimes I am distracted for a multitude of reasons; I've tired myself out too much, lack of interest, resentment to having to re-learn, or just due to healing that is taking place, or thinking of other things present, past and future.

Due to frail and erratic management of thought processes, I feel my character has changed considerably. I valued, above all, the ability to empathise and listen to other person's problems and give them some encouragement and aid. Nowadays, I cannot get my own thoughts together, for even trivial matters. I feel more self-centered in a conversation because if I do not deliver my thoughts on the spur of the moment, I have forgotten what I originally wanted to say. I might possibly use the wrong, inaccurate words, which put a different shade of meaning on the matter. One day, I honestly felt as though I had reverted to infant-like behaviour, which was not intentional. I tried to describe an event to an aunt and the words failed me at one point, and I was sitting on the floor like a baby, head down, fingers combing the carpet, searching for the words.

A burning question for me is when will I have reached the plateau, and when must I then adjust to a new life, horizons? Only time will tell, I guess. I do believe that our emotional attitude to whatever that may be, can actually propell progress. I **loved** learning the Spanish language and did not loose it entirely, even in the first days of dysphasia, I could speak just as much Spanish. (I still have to work on Spanish). I hope I can re-train my mind again, and loose that general disorientated feeling.

In the earliest phase of dysphasia, other strangers were possibly bewildered by my turn of phrase, they could have taken me for a foreigner in my own country. Family and friends no longer detect deficiency in self-expression and articulation, perhaps the unusual pausing. The overriding problem of mines is listening and catching other people's ideas and thoughts etc. properly. I still forget a great deal, and understandably, people do tire of having to repeat themselves.

Going to the speech therapist in the later stages of dysphasia is very beneficial to know if I am going in the right direction, someone who offers a guiding hand and is very encouraging. The speech therapist is almost about the only one who is aware of my pitfalls and gives me a professionalist feed-back on my progress and often puts me back on the right track, mentally and psychologically. I feel that if people who have suffered, or are still persevering with dysphasia, could share their hope. (I fully appreciate the multiplicity and complexity of brain damage.) That tangible hope may urge, impulse others to take on the challenge in their midst and be successful too. For me, giving up reminds me of withering and decomposing leaves, branches, trunk and fruit.

Maria
(25 years old)

It is quite a thing suddenly to be deprived of the capacity for arranging letters and words, both written and spoken. It was not a physical handicap but a mental one.

   My hand was able and willing to write, but my brain could not transmit the message, with the result that I could not spell my own name.

   This dialogue can be imagined:

HAND - I'm waiting
BRAIN - R-I-H-C-R-A-D
HAND - Doesn't look right to me.
BRAIN - Wait a minute. C-H. How's that?
HAND - That looks better RICH
BRAIN - We'll leave that. Next name T-U-R-H-T
HAND - That doesn't look like me at all. Am I "me" or somebody else?
BRAIN - I'm sure it ends with T-O-N.

THE EXPERIENCE OF APHASIA

    HAND - You must do better than that!
    BRAIN - I'm tired of you. I'll try tongue.
    TONGUE - I'm ready when you are.
    BRAIN - How are receiving me? I say "Richard Thurston Bailey".
    TONGUE - That sounds like me.
    BRAIN - Where do you live?
    TONGUE - "Vine", I mean "Nine", Potsherd Screech. Look Brain, you're getting me confused ....

After a few days of tedious practice I was able to write and say my name and address. Simple sentences followed. Small sounds such as auxiliaries, prepositions or negatives gave trouble, and appeared in the wrong order, or got lost altogether.

    Large words as in the sentence "altogether". would not come right, and a dictionary did not help much as I could not find the first letter.

    My brain could receive and comprehend the spoken word, and could listen to radio. The written word penetrated more slowly, and comprehension quickly tired and attention wandered. Reading bored and tired me.

Richard Bailey
(Six months after a stroke.)

JUMBLY WORDS

A piece of free writing written by Mr. Bailey two months later ....

Fishbourne to Dell Quay and Apuldrum

There is a pleasant walk within a mile of Chichester - from Fishbourne Church to Dell Quay. There is a convenient car-park at Fishbourne Church, which is just off the by-pass, with an entrance in Apuldram Lane. The distance of the walk is three miles, and only half a mile is on the road.

From the churchyard turn to the left in a southerly direction, cross a stile in a hedge and continue by a well-trodden path straight across a field, which generally has corn in the summer.

At the far end a stile brings you to the path along the sea wall, crossing one on the mouths of the Lavant course. This stretch of the wall is a good place for observing seabirds and waders. At low water there are usually large numbers of swans, shelduck and curlew. The path crosses the outfall from the sewage works, euphemistically called "the treatment plant" where there is always a gathering of little gulls.

After the pastures, the path continues on the sea wall, passing saltings and mudberths with craft in various states of disrepair to Dell Quay. This is a place worth halting at with its ancient building on the jetty, its view down the harbour to Birdham and the waterside pub - The Crown and Anchor.

Now you have to follow the road. Across a field on the left is a picturesque group of ilexes surrounding Apuldram Farm. Turn to the left into Apuldram Lane, whose name is spelt differently at each end. Apuldram Farm are rose growers and there are several acres under roses in summer, and rows of Daffodils in spring.

Turn left outside an ancient house called "Rymans", whose garden is open a few times a year; in a hundred yards follow the path to the church. One

THE EXPERIENCE OF APHASIA

wonders how such a remote church, only a mile from Fishbourne Church, could find a congregation to fill it. No wonder it was called "silly (meaning holy) Sussex", with its plethora of small churches. The church has a fine, steeply sloping tile roof, whose eaves reach nearly six feet from the ground. In the churchyard is a splendid Plain tree.

Leave by the path skiring the field towards the harbour, through a wicket-gate and rejoin the path by which you came to Dell Quay and so retrace your steps to Fishbourne.

Richard Bailey

Saturday, 27th December, 1979, was a bright sunny day. Of course, the days after Christmas and before New Year tend to be dreary and slightly depressing - the Poet called it the "Burnt out ends of smokey days". On T.V. I watched the racing at Newbury and then walked along the river to Kingston. The Mallards, Coots and Geese look out for people with paper-bags.

I got home at about five and heard the football results on the radio. Pat was busy in the kitchen preparing tea. I said "You know, I have a rotten headache". She said "Perhaps you are sickening for 'flu, why not lie down for a while". Although I was in a muddled state I thought to myself, I don't think this is an ordinary headache. During the night I could only walk by holding the walls. Pat became alarmed when I started talking nonsense using mixed up words which were senseless, and early Sunday morning she telephoned for the Doctor. Have you noticed these crises often happen on Sundays? Later, Pat told me that the Doctor thought I had suffered a Stroke. How right he was!

JUMBLY WORDS

I to Kingston hospital and was transferred to the Atkinson Morley for tests and then back to Kingston. I could walk now and use my hand although the leg and arm were very stiff, but my speech was still mixed up, a jargon of my own, and no-one understood much of what I was saying. surely I thought, like a bad dose of 'flu, my speech will come back! The Doctors at the hospital were unable to predict what degree of recovery I might make nor how long it would be.

Some seven years later, thanks to the constant help and encouragement of the Speech Therapists, the Candidate has passed 75% but his dictation, spelling, etc., must be improved to pass for "first-honours". So, put down the paper for twenty minutes and do some work. How do you spell Chrysanthemum? Crisan .... no, start again .... Chris ....

Terry Dorsett
December 1986

It was very difficult because not having been in the situation before I tried to read expressions on his face. I tried to take ... for instance ... I heard a nurse say to him once "squeeze twice for yes and once for no"; and we tried that for a couple of days. That seemed to work. Then he started to nod and shake his head. Then one or two words came such as "No" and "Yes". He could say "Nurse" by the time he left. But apart from that there was no speech whatsoever.

Now, if any bills come in he gets the cheque book, signs the cheque, and then he tells me what to do. He's always been very tidy minded, and he's got a file that he keeps his papers in. He always turns to the right file and

THE EXPERIENCE OF APHASIA

he shows me exactly where to put the receipts. But he's more or less taken over the financial side again. He just leaves the actual filling in of the cheques to me.

Anon.
Wife of a stroke patient.

It was Easter Monday 1985 when I was getting ready for lunch. I had some friends coming, when I went outside to the greenhouse, what for, I dont know, but on entering the house I felt I was going to faint. I looked for a seat meaning to sit down for a minute, but unfortuaaly didnt make it.

Nick, my son, soon found me, and though I lapsed into unconsciouness, my mind was "with it" now and then when I was conscious, that I had a stroke. My right arm and leg would'nt move and I had lost my voice. I was 75 and had a pacemaker 5 years ago and I felt I felt that the effort it was going to cost me to talk and make myself understood, a cripple, I could not sign my own name, in fact I forgot what my name was, my mind was clear but I couldnt spell my own name, and when I learned that the rest of my life was to spent learning to talk (and that I would always stutter and stumble though my words) well I laughed and laughed, it was the only sound I could make that came out in the right way, I was 17 years in the Drama Group, I had been in several Church choirs all my life, what was their to do except laugh.

My singing voice is quite alright (if slighted cracked) I could sing before I could talk, but it when I think of what I've lost, I could read the lessons in Church without a microphone, so that it could heard in the back of the church.

JUMBLY WORDS

I have learned to talk after a fashion, I type with two fingers, with a dictionary at the ready, it takes a long time to type as I have to look up the ordinary words like unto and through.

On mature thoughts, and now 77 years old, I still think it wou have been nice if they had let me go, all the visits to hospitals, the speech therapy could have gone to younger people, after all I get older every day and sooner or later I will have to depend more on my family (thought not as yet, I dont use the hospital bus, I still go by public transport if there is no-one to drive me me there by car).

Mary Van Wyke
December 1986

Three months before
I have this stroke
I was not able to make
a full sentence.

After that I lost my
speech and taste.
Everything was backwards.

Not after helping us with Fiona and Janet
at the clinic I am much better.

Susan Butler
December 1986

THE EXPERIENCE OF APHASIA

It all begun on a Saturday morning, three years ago almost to the day. That memory of mine has chosen to be even more selective than usual and will only allow me to recall a moment or two of the journey in an ambulance on my way to hospital.

The only recall of the next few weeks is the reprehensible behavior of my next bed neighbor and how I had been in comparison.

Thats my version and I have chosen to forget a young nurse accidently recalling, a few weeks later, that the neighbor had been the gentleman, not me.

As I was to be a long term patient compared to the others a seperate ward was allocated. Steady progress was made on all fronts and vague recollections are made of my progress with reading and writing but the massive nature of the problem gradually revealed itself to me.

This was in good company as others soon revealed themselves such as the loss of right hand vision in both eyes and a massive right side stroke. Apparentley quite seperately one medical specialist detected the early stages of a rapidly developing skin cancer on the left side. This demands instant treatment and during checks a week aterwards further surgery was found to be necessary. As little pain was felt it was difficult for me to understand why the medical staff seemed so greatly concerned about it. Their concern is now clear; and I have much to be thankful for. It was two months from the beginning of it all before I was sent home.

As the weeks passed two problems became apparent reading and writing first then walking.

It was assumed by me that any difficulties with reading and writing were manifestations of the same problem but in due time it was clear to me that they had seperate involvements.

The first step on the long road to recovery of reading was to determin which of the jumble of shapes were letters or numbers and which were nothing in particular. It was apparent that they were revealed to me at any of the 360 degrees of a full circle. There was quite a struggle persuading them all to appear the same way up. Letters revealed their true function first but the ends of words are reluctant to reveal themselves even now sometimes and still quite often numbers are confused with letters. The steady progress led me to comprehend the construction of words. First the two letter and then the three letter words. Next I was taught to read longer words by systematicaly grouping 2-3 letters to construct the longer words. The five to seven letter words are still generally the greatest problem as longer words seem to reveal themselves more readily. Another problem is that words reveal shemselves more readily as components of a phrase than as individual words.

Writing recovered rapidly but three years later reading is still only progressing slowly. This progress has only been possible by the help of the speech therapists and recently by the help of others at a local education centre.

Walking has also slowly improved with the help from the Local Mobility Officers and I shall soon be learning to cook and look after myself.

There is much to be thankful for in the dedicated help given to me by others. Perhaps the one who has given the most dedicated help to me is my wife who has problems of her own to deal with. My thanks to her were expressed by asking her to join me at a celebration visit to St Martins-in-the-Field followed by a visit to the National Art Gallery and a celebration lunch.

THE EXPERIENCE OF APHASIA

These three sketches are selected from those I have drawn over the last three years to show the recovery I have made with the help of friends in the Art Club to recover my former skills.

Mr. D. Mott.

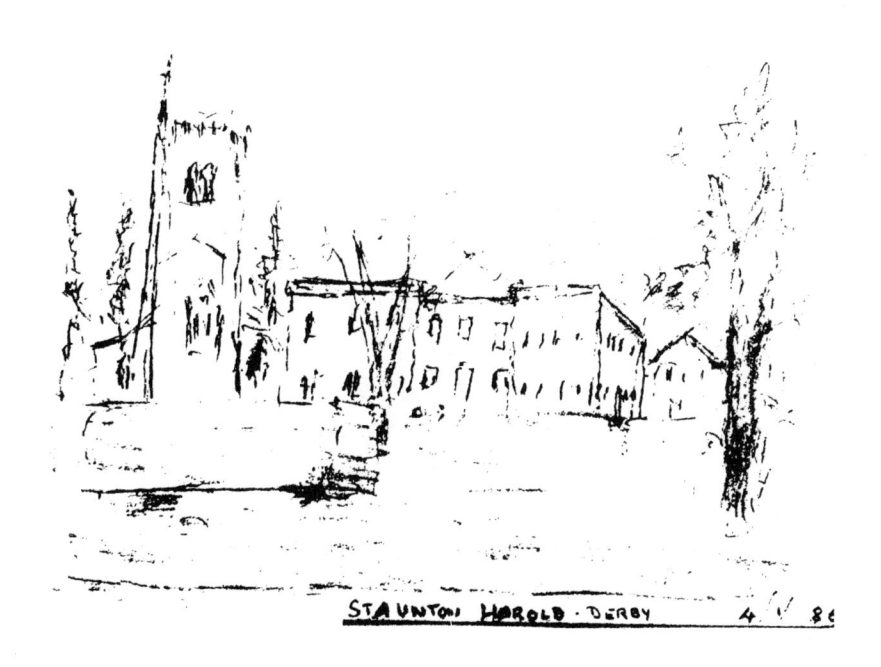

JUMBLY WORDS

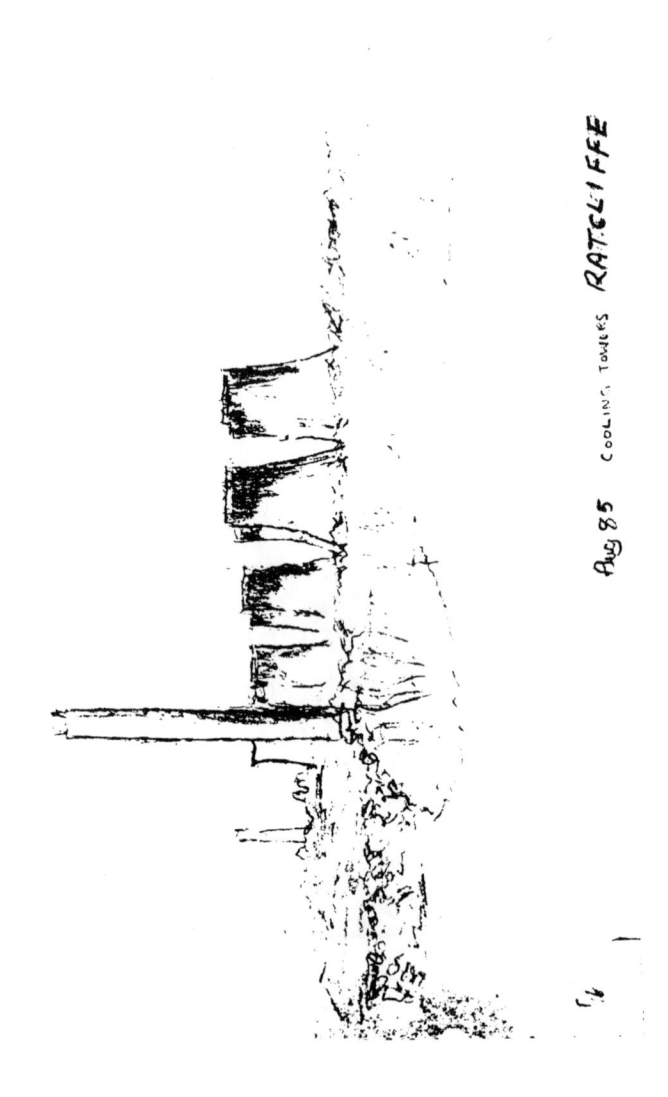

THE EXPERIENCE OF APHASIA

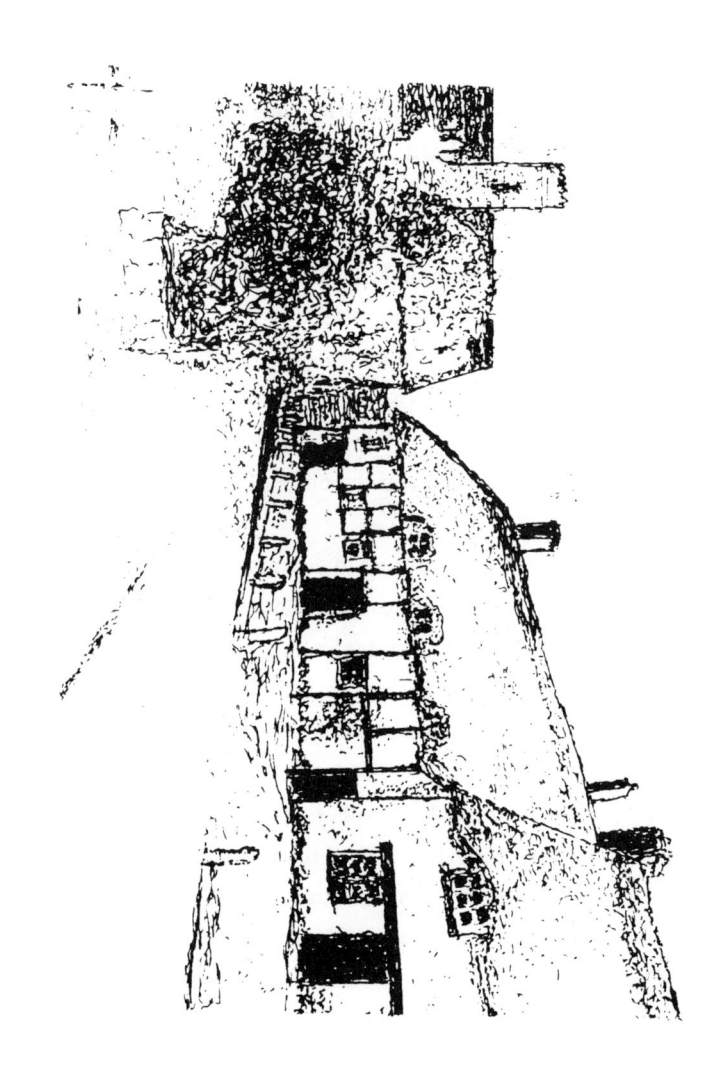

JUMBLY WORDS

Transcript of a Tape Recording Made by a Speech Therapist

Speech Therapist: Can we talk again about when you were first ill. Tell me again about that first Thursday.

Mr. H.: Well I was busy collecting the papers to give in the shop. It was like an explosion in my head to start with. But I put it off and the following week I went to see the doctor and my blood pressure was quite high, and she had made an arrangement for me to go into hospital, and the doctor there said to me he thought I'd had a slight stroke, and they sent me home and that was when the other attack happened, that was the Thursday June 25th. It happened in the back garden. I collapsed and I couldn't get up, and eventually my wife phoned the doctor and she came out, and she got me into Casualty that night. I don't have very much recollection of that.

Speech Therapist: When do you remember first noticing other people did not understand you?

Mr. H.: I think when I was trying to communicate with my wife at home. I don't know what - the doctor seemed to make out that I was trying to ask for food and I had difficulty communicating that to my wife. I hadn't eaten all day and I wanted some food before I went to hospital. The speech had gone away with the first attack and come back again remarkably enough - back to normal, but after that second attack it completely went, and I had difficulty even understanding other people, and I had difficulty communicating with other folk. It's a bit vague about that time.

Speech Therapist: Do you remember what your feelings were about that?

Mr. H.: I think, as far as I can recall, I had a couldn't care less attitude about the whole thing. I think it was the fact it was nature's way of doing for me to reduce my blood pressure. I wasn't really caring a damn, in fact, my wife said to me laterally in the hospital I couldn't have given a damn. Even when she came to visit me it was first like visiting a stranger. I was in another world really. It's very difficult to describe. It was like being on another planet. And it was when I went back to the second hospital. That's when I started to pick up. And I was very determined to get back to good health again. That's when I concentrated mostly on my speech. And I was very determined from then on.

Speech Therapist: Do you remember having speech therapy when you were in hospital?

Mr. H.: Yes, I had a couple of visits and my performance was very poor as far as I can recollect.

Speech Terapist: Do you remember what you felt about that?

Mr. H.: At that time in hospital I don't think it troubled me particularly. I don't know. I seemed to have a "couldn't care less" attitude to it - to everything.

Speech Therapist: How did you feel when you got home?

Mr. H.: Well I was delighted to get home. And I think all my thoughts were concentrated on getting things right - particularly the voice.

Speech Therapist: How do you mean, your voice?

Mr. H.: Well I wanted to communicate. Before I had been writing things down in order to communicate with my wife and sons.

Speech Therapist: So was your writing better than your speaking?

Mr. H.: Yes, at this stage. It was a bit garbled to start with, but latterly it wasn't too bad, but it was words of almost one syllable. I just couldn't make myself understood to anybody. I think when I got out of hospital the speech wasn't really very good at that stage - looking back.

Speech Therapist: When did you start to be concerned about it? When did you lose the "couldn't care less" attitude?

Mr. H.: When I went back to the second hospital latterly. I somehow communicated with my wife over the phone - I don't know how I did it - and I said "Bring my clothes in", and I think that was the kind of step forward. I said "Bring my clothes in" and that was me determined to get better. Up until then I couldn't have cared less. That was the turning point I think.

Speech Therapist: How difficult was it for you when you got home?

Mr. H.: It was very difficult to start with, in fact it was very difficult, and very traumatic for all concerned.

Speech Therapist: What kind of effect do you think it had on your family?

Mr. H.: I'm trying to think. Well, the boys were very understanding. All of them I suppose. My oldest boy when he came home - because he'd been away for some months after my illness, and he's less understanding than his brother because he lived through it and lived with me.

Speech Therapist: What kind of worries did you have about it when you came home, about the business and so on?

Mr. H.: Well I was very concerned, in fact I was thinking about selling the business at one stage, because my wife was having such problems running the business, and I couldn't do anything to help her, but things have got better and better as time has gone on. So things aren't too bad now but my wife says I'm still impossible to live with at times.

Speech Therapist: In what ways do you think you are difficult to live with?

Mr. H.: I think I've got a very short fuse. That's the sum and substance of it. I flare up very, very easily and for no reason at all, and I'm trying to control that to the best of my ability. Almost to the extent I leave it to them, and if I know it's an argument I should be involved with, I tend to step back from it, and let them get on with it, because it doesn't do me any good and it doesn't do anybody any good.

Speech Therapist: What did it feel like when you realised you had difficulty reading and writing and counting?

Mr. H.: I think the most shock was when I discovered I couldn't count cash - the denominations and so on, and that came as a bit of a shock to

THE EXPERIENCE OF APHASIA

me, and that was rather traumatic. I had been warned about the other aspect of my difficulty, but I'd never been warned I couldn't count cash after a lifetime of counting cash and that was traumatic. The rest I was well warned and I just took in my stride. But I used to be able to write most fluently and the brain and the pen were as one, but now it takes thought. Now you've got to think about it and it's the same with speech. It used to be automatic. Now the word escapes me. The Key word. I was talking to a man yesterday and I said "Just a minute", and the word eventually came to me. I am amazed at normal people - how they can mix up the words.

Speech Therapist: What kind of reactions did you get from other people - other than your own family?

Mr. H. Well, people basically were most surprised that I was able to communicate at that time, and they were pleased for me. People in my walk of life, mostly friends and customers knew the set up and when I met someone I tended to let them know I had an impediment in my speech, either that, or that I'd had a stroke, and that put them at their ease. So it was difficult for people I didn't know, but the majority of people I came across knew my problem and people have been very kind and very understanding. It's never presented much of a difficulty for me throughout the illness. I've always had a go, no matter what my speech has been like.

Speech Therapist: Do you remember you went on holiday quite soon after you came out of hospital? What do you remember about your talking at that time?

Mr. H. Well, it wasn't so good. I just remember we were in company and I never let them know, and I felt a bit out of it because my wife was talking to the assembled company and I wasn't communicating with them at all, but if I'd let them know at the time about my difficulty it would probably have been a lot easier. I felt a bit out of it then, but that's the only time.

I think I felt rotten about it - the lack of communication. In fact, I was talking to the barman earlier in the evening and I told him my problem, and it was much easier after that. People tend to get embarrassed. I was never embarrassed but people tend to get embarrassed, but it never bother me that way.

Speech Therapist: What about some of the particular problems you have had - like your wife commented that your voice was too loud?

Mr. H.: Well I think as far as I'm concerned, I take criticism very badly, but the point of the matter was, I wasn't aware my voice was so loud, and I was so conscious of concentrating on speaking, I lost sight of the fact the sound was very much more than it had been before, so I've modulated that since then, and I think it's been quite an improvement. But that's another thing, I take it very personally even if I'm not being criticised, if people are not criticising me, I tend to flare up at that and that's a thing I've got to watch, whenever I'm criticised, even although it's constructive criticism I tend to flare up, but I think it's all part of the same syndrome.

Speech Therapist: What are your hopes for the future?

Mr. H. Well, I hope to get back to normal. It's nearly back to normal as far as I'm concerned and it's just a question of convincing yourself. My health's a lot better now. I'm working in the shop more often. I don't think I'll ever get back to normal as before, but I'll as near as damn it to what I was before, and that's my self-determination, and as far as I'm concerned I would hope to be back to as near as normal in the not too distant future. My wife tells me I talk on - even in the early days when she didn't understand me. My wife says "You're always blethering to folk." There's only one way .... on and on.

Peter Heywood and Speech Therapist
February 1987

Chapter 6

THE FUTURE

"... has the brain already reached the utmost of its healing? ...... Ay, there's the rub."

One man's feelings about his minimal dysphasia

It is with some trepidation, that I write, as fully as I can, some of the problems that beset me. These of course can be real, as in the case of lack of dexterity in the fingers of my right hand; where the sense of touch is diminished. The right arm too has suffered from what I believe is called a frozen shoulder.

Then there are the imaginary doubts as to my future. If a typist didn't find work for two years, she would know that on returning to work she would find her typing was slower, but with practise would soon return to her normal speed.

For me this no longer holds true, as a result of the brain damage I sustained. I feel that shuld I return to doing my previous type of work, not only would I be totally unaware of my function, but would I retain my previous expertise, or would I be able to do the work at all.

People and friends tell me that in conversation they would not be aware that I had any problems, but this is only when speaking in general conversation. When I come to using the telephone, I can always remember a name, but find it exceedingly difficult to remember the gist of a conversation on the phone, or to remember what number to call on. This is probably the result of a strange voice and the gaps in being able to memorise more than two instructions.

My writing attemps give rise for grave concern, plus the gaps in my memory regarding vocabulary. I have been working hard as possible on trying to rectify these inadequacies. My Speech Therapist tells me how well I have done. I know within my own limits what I am capable of, and am aware that my faculties are at least forty per cent under par.

In the ability to learn, I too find problems. My wife is helping me to read my tables, this for a man who knew quadratics, loci, trignometry to vector j. This is an area which has diminished beyond reason, and so back to the drawing board, and calls for a great amount of revision on mathematics, radio theory, chemistry and physics.

The ability to read clearly is there, but to a lesser degree than before. I find it very difficult now to realy get into a book, and frequently now give up, mainly out of sheer boredom.

At the moment my stamps, stamp album, catalogues, letters from the Stamp Club and price lists from in stamps, occupy the greater part of my time, that and helping in my and my mother's gardens, takes up a lot of time. Now with the weather as it has been, there is little hope of gardening activities.

The lack of memory, problems in expressing matters concisely and to the point, places my future in an invidious position. I see no future at all at the moment, but there is still that caustic something that tells me to keep trying.

Another of my problems is my own lack of confidence; which by now has been whittled to non-existence. It is easy not to feel this, if your prospects to find work are good. But what can be done for a forty three year old man, who has been out of work for some two and a half years - it is at this point that failure tends to rear its head.

Such are my inabilities, I find it hard to correspond with the knowledge

THE EXPERIENCE OF APHASIA

that my words may not be incisive or to the point. There is little I can do about this. For me it has been an endless struggle to get even this far along the path to recovery. This is no futile attempt believe me, I will have this brain of mine working to its true capacity if it takes another five years, but the frustration, anger and demoralising attributes comes home with the overwhelming wish that perhaps it would be better if I lived in that grey world I was subject to during the time of the brain damage.

Mr. B.M.

Nineteen Eighty One when I had my haemorrhage I was thirty two years old.

I felt that it was only a temporary thing, about six weeks. I couldn't understand why I couldn't speak. I didn't realise until later that I coudn't compunicate.

I rember they put the cot side up to stop me getting out. I rember I wanted to get out to go to the loo.

Now six years later I have two boys aged five years and three years. I look after the yougest as my wife works as a teacher. The eldest is at school nine in the morning to twelve, then I take him home for lunch and return him to school in the afternoon.

As part of my rehabitation I became involved with aking stools, just general activity cooking and cleaning. I also started carpentry. I made my own coffee table. I also finished two dawers bed storage spaces and toy bod.

Last summer I relandscaped the garden, I have also made a dark room for photography. I develope my film and then print them. I now drive the car after being classed "fit".

Inspited of all that I can do there are times when I wish this had not happened. However I am glad I did not die.

M. Hopirott

From the very beginning the inability to speak was a crushing blow and the more because I could not explain my fears and bewilderments of my situation.

At the beginning my memory of what I could say is not very clear, but it was very little and that ill-pronounced. So it was then the Speech Therapist entered my life. I had not gone into hospital and so I missed the "picking up" procedure which takes place there. The result was, through nobodys fault, that I missed the first two to three weeks.

She visited me at home, and filled me with such hope that it remains with me to this day. It was not only her professionalism which struck me, was the sincere dedication with which she applied, and the kindness and sympathy that was evident. From the very first she filled me with confidence and that has given me the will to work.

She tested me to see what I was able to do and she found the results abysmally poor. At this time she was seeing me twice a week, giving vowel sound and voiced and voiceless sounds. Later on she gave tongue and lip exercises. About this time I was experiencing the health problems, so I felt I was not making headway.

She took me across to a Christmas Party given by the Chest, Heart and Stroke Association, but I not have a word to say. After Christmas I began seeing her at the Hospital every Friday and it was from then that the systematic work was begun.

If the lessons had a format which could be described it would be as follows: conversation, solving pronunciation difficulties which I brought to the lesson, specific occasions causing difficulty, exercises and new activities. But furthermore there was a good understanding friend that was prepared to listen no matter what the subject was about. There was method in the madness.

Innumerable aids were used: the P.T.M. Cards and Books: recognition of various things, household objects and the like: building sentences from a picture, describing a picture, building up a story from pictures given; logicality exercises; giving and following instruction; nouns verbs, tenses from pictures given. These are only a very sample from material provided and those which she prepared. Then there were tape recordings I would make, and criticism and analysis to follow.

After Christmas I was introduced to the Group Therapy Class which met every Wednesday. To begin with I was perplexed. I was expecting everyone to be like me but I began to find that every stroke is different. The majority could speak better than I could, but many had infirmities which I did not have. Some could speak perfectly, but could understand little. Gradually I came to value the fellowship which I found there and discovered a real co-operation and friendship amongst them. It was then I realised I had to give as well as to receive. There was an idea with me that stroke patients are always kindly disposed and accept their burden cheerfully.

She has done a splendid job, as indeed the other speech therapists have done. She has built a confidence which has enabled me to take my part in company once again. A point was made that I did not look to the future, long and full of hard work, but I looked back and saw the successes and built on them.

And so I look forward to the future knowing the limitations, but full of confidence. I look back on the nights I was awake in the small hours wondering if I would ever make the personal of "I" ever again. Many is the hours when I tried it without success.

By dint of hard work and moderate success, I have beated into the background that another stroke much worse, and possibly fatal, might occur. I live today, confidentally, that the next month will be so much better than the last month.

As I go on improving, the more difficulties happen. When I could speak only a little, the mind wasn't alert then and no problem was encountered, but now I can speak any word at all, with some difficulty perhaps my voice is in danger of running ahead of myself.

My recall of words, my seeking to clothe my ideas in words and my wanting to express ideas in the wealth of words as I used to, is causing frustration. My mind, so to speak, is in advance of my brain.

How to come to terms with these problems? My speech therapist has discussed the matter with me and has led the way with constructive plans. But nevertheless the brain still lags behind with providing the words that one needs in conversation.

What is one to do? One must keep working away at the contingency plans eg. circumlocute, synonyms, and so on. One must keep listing the words found as stumbling blocks, completing crosswords, playing scrabble and keeping the diary; indeed every way one knows to keep words alive and to keep recall ever-advancing.

But the one question that is always being asked is, "Has the brain already reached the utmost of its healing?"

Ay, there's the rub.

John Hughes

THE EXPERIENCE OF APHASIA

After I had a Stroke it was difficult to judge whether I could work again. My Company were very good and kept me on full salary for a year. My speech was very poor and I couldn't recite the Alphabet. With the help of the Speech Therapists I tried to do as much work as I could on speech exercises and recording and listening to my voice on the tape recorder.

In the Spring of 1980 I went once a week to a Rehabilitation Unit. This was a very low time for me. I was able to talk a little but was in a group of peole who could converse readily. However, they are physically handicapped. The stroke patient feels very isolated and emotion and depression are always close to the surface.

In January 1981 I was lucky to get a place at a Dysphasia Centre where ninety per cent of the patients had suffered a stroke. At that time it was obvious I could not go back to my job and the Company retired me with a pension. As it happened, they were "taken-over" within two years and I would probably have been made redundant anyway.

My speech etc., slowly improved. However, my own experience of the Centre was that it was not everyones "cup of tea" particularly when the patient's character tended to be introverted. There were times when I didn't want to go at all.

In October 1983 I went back to the Rehabilitation Unit and saw the Psychologist who gave me some tests in order to make an up-to-date assessment of my capabilities. I found the tests frustrating as it was impossible for me to remember three numbers or letters at a time after a matter of seconds. This was put down to loss of short-term memory.

I was surprised and rather disappointed to learn that there was not a work Register for handicapped people of firms willing to employ such people. I imagine the patient who has had a nervous breakdown or someone recently out of prison feels the same. The younger stroke patient probably would like to feel there is a chance of a small job, at least on a part-time basis. Of course, the employment position is not good particularly in the commercial world where things change very quickly.

Should a patient have to go to a Rehabilitation Unit for four consecutive days in order to be re-assessed?

Terry Dorsett
December 1986

Tomorrow, I hope, Dr. ____ will confirm that I can return to work as an out-patient. I will have been on sick leave for 12 weeks! It's interesting to speculate concerning that time.

The recovery has been like a number of steps - sometimes it would be two or three weeks when there would be no discernable improvement, then there would be a spectacular bound. For example, I happened to awaken two nights in succession when a friend came home late - on the first I babbled almost incoherently, on the second, almost normal.

I have noticed the necessity to talk with people - in a queue for example. Up to a week or so ago, I would have carefully considered what I would say but now I say what ordinary words come forth. I happened to sit with a lady (a stranger in fact) at a dinner for nearly an hour; at the end I explained about the stroke and she assured me that there was no suggestion ever of a hesitation in my voice - very encouraging!

I note with interest what I imagine my colleagues will say during the first few days - I think they will all start off with good wishes and will then come straight to the point!

THE EXPERIENCE OF APHASIA

I feel very much better now and I feel confident to tackle the work of a Headmaster. I'm aware that I am going to be tired at times during the day, but I have every intention of relaxing if it's only for a moment or two.

John
3 months after a stroke.

I was fifty-four years old, my husband Tom, fifty-eight, we were a normal couple with varied interests outside our work and home.

On the morning of the 14th March we both went off to work as usual. This was the last time for many months we would be able to say this again.

My husband was brought home from work feeling unwell; our Doctor diagnosed a mild stroke, but after three days Tom could not speak at all and was admitted to hospital. Now my nightmare really began. How would I cope with someone who couldn't speak? One day I'd a healthy, outgoing husband, the next - one who couldn't speak, raise his right arm or leg, or look at all like himself.

After a few sleepless nights I thought to myself "Get on with it - it is not going to help feeling sorry for yourself and it won't help Tom".

From that day I was determined I would help him in every way to regain his confidence and return to as near normality as we could.

Within a few days, with the help of the speech therapists, Tom could say "yes" and "no". Quite an achievement, believe me! I felt so proud of him. Two whole words! After four weeks in hospital he was allowed home. He was determined to perfect his speech and worked at it very hard, despite being overcome with extreme tiredness after the least physical or mental effort.

JUMBLY WORDS

At this time his speech was still very limited.

The most difficult thing to cope with was his quick temper. This was in complete contrast to his former personality. Shaving, dressing, moving round the house - all these things took much longer to achieve. Driving the car was out all together and this was one thing he really enjoyed previously. All these things may seem unimportant but they are, when you have known the person concerned to be very capable prior to his stroke.

I have often wondered if life will ever return to normal, and I feel very guilty and selfish to feel this. No-one knows the uphill struggle both the patient and relatives have, to achieve even the slightest improvement.

Information on how to help the stroke victim is not readily available. I feel hospitals could help by giving the relatives some guidance by way of leaflets etc. I found out from newspaper ads. and wrote to the Chest, Heart and Stroke Association for leaflets, read them and started from there to attack the problem. No way were we giving in!

My husband was lucky and had the help of speech therapists three days per week. In between, we worked together to improve his speaking, reading and writing, by repeated practice, again and again and again. I noticed a marked improvement when we were in company. It was as if he played to the audience. He seemed stimulated by company, so out we went on a more regular basis.

Tom's confidence grew and his speech got gradually better. I found it helped to be able to laugh at some of our problems, like the day it took him an hour to tell me he'd had a visitor. It was like a guessing game with clues, but we eventually succeeded. "The Minister" was the answer.

Now after eleven months working together we have achieved something. My husband can converse reasonably well, doesn't get stuck for words as often, and recognises when he is being unreasonable.

THE EXPERIENCE OF APHASIA

We go swimming, walking, to the theatre, out for meals, visiting and entertaining friends. No way can any of these things be done as well as before, but at least we are making progress.

Maybe in another eleven months, no one will ever know that our lives were turned upside down by the results of a stroke.

Laura

The first week I had no recollection of happenings at all. The second week, I remember speech therapists and physiotherapists visiting the ward. Physiotherapists helped greatly by showing how to cope with leg and arm movements. Speech therapists tried to make me say one syllable words.

Ward staff were very helpful, insisting that I had to ask for tea, sugar and milk. At this stage, even saying one word, yes or no, was a most major effort, after which I was very tired. Obviously the great effort to concentrate was exhausting.

After coming home from hospital I returned for speech therapy three times per week. After a short period of physiotherapy my physical disability was vastly improved. Speech, however, was another problem. After each speech therapy session I was physically drained, but after approximately six weeks I could string a few words together to make myself understood, but still was having great difficulty forming words. I knew what I wanted to say but I couldn't get it out.

I found that I could remember most things but still had this frustrating inability to communicate.

JUMBLY WORDS

As well as speech difficulties I was experiencing great difficulty with the basic three R's, trying to control the pen and write, even my name, entailed great mental and physical strain. After achieving this I would be most disappointed at the results. Even yet after ten months, my writing does not bear a great deal of resemblance to my former hand.

I had to prove to myself that I could still meet and talk to people. I was out of hospital one week when I went to the Fiddler's Rally with my wife and four friends, who all understood my problems. Strange as it may seem I found it very easy to sing along with the band - much easier than speaking. We went to a hotel for drinks and coffee and I felt I had made my very first contact with the social scene again, albeit more restrained than before.

My next step was to continue my association with Scouting, where I had been Chairman of the district. During my weeks in hospital all my friends in scouting had kept in touch and I did not find it too difficult to attend the Annual General Meeting for my district, in spite of my intention to relinquish my position as chairman at this time. I did not feel fluent enough to continue. I do intend, if improvement continues, to renew my involvement in scouting.

Every day, weather permitting, I forced myself to go out walking, increasing the length of my walks daily. This also helped me to speak to acquaintances, and also helped my physical fitness, giving me another interest outside the four walls.

After ten months I now feel able to cope with most social functions. I find I can think more for myself regarding simple household duties e.g. preparing a meal, washing up - something I couldn't cope with at all, at the beginning.

I'm much slower at all these things but I can at least accomplish them at my own pace now.

THE EXPERIENCE OF APHASIA

I would like to think that in another six months my improvement will continue and I will be able to fulfill a useful purpose in life again.

Tom

Looking back over the last nearly ten years, I was nothing but a cabbage with a wandering mind, no great pain at that time, a stroke sufferer, quite dumb. The pain came later. Now I forget the suffering; I lead a very busy life, transported around the house in a wheelchair, endeavouring to fit everything in that has to be done that day. My speech is nowhere near perfect and will never be; I have to miss half the words through the rapid way that all folk do; that is Dysphasia which follows with many stroke cases; I was one of the unlucky ones. But I am certainly no cabbage.

I am no doctor, no neuro-surgeon, just a very ordinary person who talks straight from a stroke-disabled body, not from a disabled mind.

To all friends who succumbed to the traumatic, life-blood sucking stroke, minor or massive, the most important advice is always the same: keep your eyes straight forward. NEVER GIVE UP, PRESS ON. It's a long, hard road to traverse, but there's always a light beyond, however dim; it grows brighter the more you push through.

I know, I have travelled the whole road right from the start. I'm still travelling, but the sun is shining and lighting my way now. May I hope that you will find the courage to traverse through the dark also to greet the sun, knowing that it *is* possible.

Arthur J. West
10 years after his stroke

JUMBLY WORDS

The Experience of Dysphasia

In one morning of late August I went to do a little light gardening. Within five minutes I found myself spreadeagled on the ground. Almost at once I staggered up into the house; in answer to my wife's anxious enquiries, I could produce only unintelligible gibberish.

That was the beginning of my stroke. The doctor sent me to bed and the following morning my speech was not improved and he sent me to hospital. There I was examined and X Rayed and they found nothing physically wrong. During the days whilst in hospital I came to realise that it was impossible to pronounce a single word.

When I lay down in the ambulance I could see only the tops of trees and houses with no guide to direction to which of four hospitals in the vicinity we were driving to. Therefore, when the following afternoon my wife came to visit, my plea of "Where am I?" was not understood and my efforts to ask this question reduced me to tears. Only a letter sent to me by a neighbour revealed the hospital's name. It was strange to me that my effort to talk to nurses and fellow-patients only brought kindly but non-comprehensive stares.

My wife on a subsequent visit was sought out by the speech therapist and arrangements were made for weekly appointments for me after discharge. After seeing the fellow members of the group, many in wheel chairs and with paralysis, I realised how fortunate I was and self-pity was dispelled.

These visits taught me to write and speak albeit from the kindergarten stage, from the time when I remembered my school-days.

During the course of about five months I have learned to write again; and hopefully to speak with increasing fluency. All this while I have been taught with patience and skill by those ladies who appoint the weekly visits. In particular I am indebted to the therapist who gives me individual

THE EXPERIENCE OF APHASIA

sessions and homework, which together have encouraged and helped greatly, without them I should have lacked motive and understanding.

I have always been a zealous reader, but now have to measure my capacity for thinking to limited spells, this applies to mental exercise and to conversation. The periods of clear thinking gradually are now extended before a headache and discomfort compels a rest.

My wife tells me that my temper is worse than ever, but I cannot argue with her as excitement renders me temporarily speechless, and leaves her with a triumphant smile.

It appears my memory of facts and figures and names is failing, but probably this is due to my age rather than dysphasia; as I am approaching my 83rd birthday.

It is obvious to me that my patience will need to be extended and also the patience of those who listen to me before fluent speech returns, if it ever does, until then nil desperandum.

John Wells
February 1987

JUMBLY WORDS

Quotations:

I have noticed the necessity to talk with people.

    John: 3 months after a stroke.

Of all the afflictions effected by a stroke I feel the loss of speech to be the most frustrating and debilitating for both patients and their spouses.

    Vera West

All you know is lieing in bed with people coming and going.

    J. E. Lyall

Confidence is the one thing omitted when they list the handicaps caused by strokes.

    Jack Hughes

THE EXPERIENCE OF APHASIA

From the beginning, the loss of speech was a crushing blow - the more because I could not explain my fears and bewilderments of my situation

    John Hughes

I seemed to have become an idiot.

    Mrs. H.

I only realised my wife was there by the feel of her wedding ring on her finger.

    Jim

Then the enormity of the catastrophe seaped through my damaged brain.

    Lily Reid

Not being able to read, write or talk is no joke.

    Monique

JUMBLY WORDS

Within a few days, with the help of speech therapists, Tom could say "yes" and "no". Quite an achievement believe me! I felt so proud of him. Two whole world.

    Laura

I don't actually believe in the Resurrection but there is something going on up there.

    John Graney

A way of life changed in a minute of time.

    Christine Bayliss
